The History of
Sikh Dharma of the
Western Hemisphere

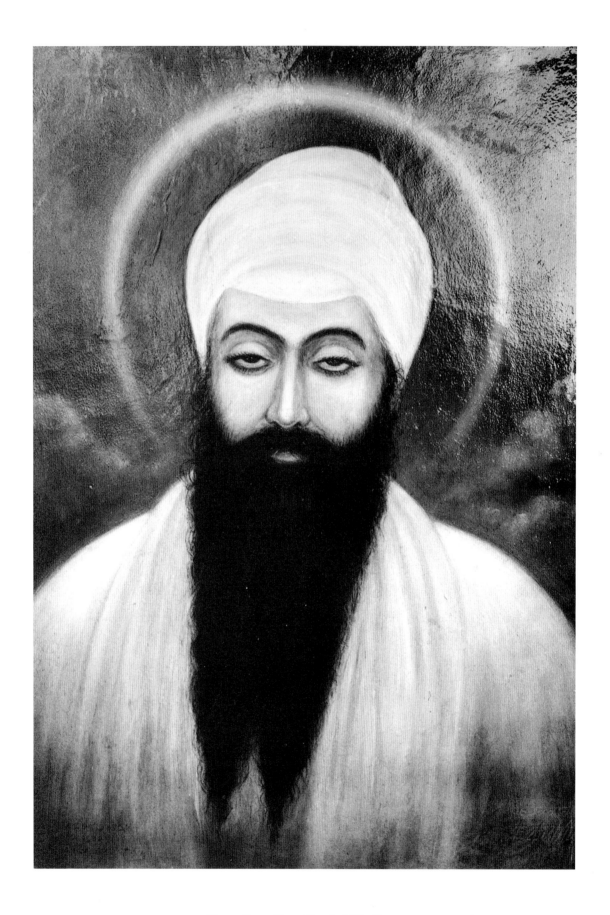

Guru Ram Das, Forth Sikh Guru

The History of Sikh Dharma of the Western Hemisphere

Text: S.S. Shanti Kaur Khalsa
Photography Editor: S.S. Soorya Kaur Khalsa

First published in 1995 by
Sikh Dharma Publications
Route 3, Box 132d
Española, N.M. 87532

Editor: S.S. Gurutej Singh Khalsa
Photography Editor: S.S. Soorya Kaur Khalsa
Design: Mary Shapiro

Front cover: The Harimandir Sahib in Amritsar. Photo: Sikh Dharma Archives
Back cover: S.S. Pritpal Singh Khalsa and his son, Sat Pal Singh Khalsa, during a visit to India in 1995.
Photo: Soorya Kaur Khalsa

Printed in Hong Kong by Colorcorp, Inc.

ISBN # 0-9639847-4-8

Contents

Dedication

To the Siri Singh Sahib whose guidance and light have ignited the fire of Guru's love in the hearts of untold millions around the world.

Foreword

Two hundred years before the dawn of the Renaissance began to shed its rays on Europe, the Bhakti movement had begun in India. Around the time a young man named Francis walked naked from the village of Assisi, saintly men in love with God walked away from the grip and control the religions of India held on the society and sang their songs of praise to the One Creator. Like St. Francis of Assisi, who was in love with God and sang to Him in his own language, rather than the language of the Church, the Bhaktis sang their songs of praise in the language of the people rather than in Sanskrit.

By the time of the Renaissance in the 14th century, there were remarkable similarities between the evolution of religious thought in Europe and in India. The dominant influence of Europe was the institution of the Church and the clergy who controlled every aspect of people's lives. The dominant influence of India was Hinduism and caste-elite Brahmins who also controlled every aspect of people's lives. The Christian scriptures were written in Latin, a little used language reserved for writing and intellectual discussions. All religious services were conducted in Latin. The language of the Hindu Brahmins was Sanskrit, another language used only for intellectual treatises and discourses.

The Bhaktis wrote and prayed in the common language of the people. What they taught and practiced was that the experience of God was within the grasp of the individual and not up to the dictates of the pundits. It is a personal evolution and, the Bhaktis taught, attainable through the continuous repetition of any of the many Names of God. *God*, in fact, is only just another Name of God.

Like the monks of Europe who kept most of the available knowledge of the time guarded in their monasteries, the Brahmins kept the wealth of India's knowledge to themselves, maintaining control over the order and evolution of Indian society. Further, the yogis and rishis of India, those ascetics who had the greatest depth of spiritual knowledge, secluded themselves in the wilderness, hiding from the world in caves and forests and frozen mountain tops.

The 14th century also brought the earliest rumblings of reform in the Church. Walter Lollard and John Huss openly preached for reform and were put to death for heresy. In India, the intolerance of the Brahmins lead to the overthrow and expulsion of Buddhism from India. Yet the 14th century also witnessed the lives of Kabir and Ramanand, two of the greatest Bhakti saints whose writings are found in the *Siri Guru Granth Sahib,* the sacred scriptures of the Sikhs.

One other prevailing influence on the evolution of religious thought in India was the aggressive introduction of Islam. The 12th century brought the first of several Muslim invaders to India and a prosperous, though elitist, Islamic society flourished. Each successive invader exceeded the intolerance and atrocities of the previous one, destroying ancient Hindu temples and putting tens of thousands of Hindus to death, mostly in cold blood. Approximately 60 foreign invasions of India took place between the 11th century and end of the 15th century, with the most destructive campaign still to come under Babar. Yet life evolved, and the sparks of the Bhakti movement that were struck in the 14th century caught fire in the 15th century.

The latter part of the 15th century was a time of sweeping changes in the world. In Europe, domination of the Church on the people was becoming unbearable to many. Superstition and fear of damnation kept the society shackled to a rigid social order few dared to challenge. The great monastic movements were at their peak, keeping knowledge and literacy secluded from the masses that desperately needed it. Those who could bring healing and relief to the world locked themselves away in the sanctity of the medieval monasteries. Great debates took place in those monasteries, not to discuss ways to relieve the suffering of the people, but to discuss how many angels could dance on a pinhead.

In India, the Brahmins dictated to a caste-bound society the sequence of their lives. Spirituality was measured by intellectual contests where sutras of various scriptures were quoted to prove meaningless points of theology. The growing fanaticism of the Muslims prevented tolerance or understanding. The yogis, who held the technology of spiritual enlightenment and relief of suffering, kept to the forests and mountains, guarding their secrets greedily. The practice of black tantra, or black magic, was prevalent and holy men were usually recognized by the magic tricks they performed.

Into this world of darkness, in 1469, 23 years before the discovery of America, came Guru Nanak, the first Sikh Guru. The impact of Guru Nanak's teachings on 15th century India was profound. The impact of his teachings on the world is still unfolding. Challenging, then changing, the religious thought that had prevailed for centuries, Guru Nanak implemented a social order based on the consciousness of the individual and the individual's sovereign right to have his own living experience of consciousness; to see God within the man and the man's conscious responsibility to the society.

In the India of Guru Nanak's day, as in medieval Europe, religious people were renunciates and survived by begging. Yet Guru Nanak taught that the life of the householder was the highest yoga, that work is a worship and, most radically for that time, that women have equal rights and an equal relationship to God with that of men.

Guru Nanak denounced the control of the Brahmins over Hindu society and discounted intellectual theology. He brought to light the esoteric rituals and caste prejudices prevalent among Hindus, teaching that all men are equal in the eyes of God and that there is no secret between God and Man. He challenged the intolerance and fanaticism of the Muslims, demonstrating that God dwells in all places and innerspaces. He chastised the yogis, secluded in their forests and caves, for failing their social responsibility to mankind by choosing a life of renunciation.

He gave only one commandment, which is *Jap*—the recitation of the Name of God. More technically, *Jap* is the practice of the individual to continually identify himself with the Universal Identity by generating within himself the identical vibrational frequency to the Cosmic vibrational frequency, and through that harmony of vibration, transform his conscious awareness to the Universal Awareness. *Jap!* Reciting those sounds that are the identity of God Himself, not only His formal Name, but His nickname as well. It is an intimate relationship between the individual, his soul, and his God.

For 22 years Guru Nanak traveled by foot across India, South Asia, and the Middle East spreading his simple message and changing the awareness of the world forever. When he finally settled down as an aging householder, it was in the Punjab region of northern India that remains today the homeland of the Sikhs. Guru Nanak was succeeded by nine other Gurus who gave the shape and identity to Sikh Dharma and set heroic examples of humility, commitment, and sacrifice.

The fifth Guru, Guru Arjun, compiled the scripture of the Sikhs, which he called the *Adi Granth*. It was composed of the writings of the previous four Gurus, plus his own, and the sacred writings of other Hindu and Muslim Bhakti saints who, in their states of ecstasy, described their experiences of consciousness and what they did to attain them. When the *Adi Granth* was completed, Guru Arjun directed that it should be translated into all languages so that "the Word of the Guru can spread across the world like oil on water." Today we see that prophecy coming true.

Then the tenth Guru, Guru Gobind Rai, did something truly unique. First he called for five of his Sikhs to offer their heads as sacrifice to their Dharma. It appeared that the Guru had gone mad and beheaded his own disciples. Yet he brought those five before the congregation, radiant and transformed. He then gave them baptism, known as Amrit. After they had taken the Amrit, Guru Gobind Rai pronounced them as Khalsa, the Brotherhood of the Pure Ones. The Guru then asked his own Sikhs to administer the Amrit to him, saying, *"Khalsa mero satgur poora."* "Khalsa is my True Guru." By taking the Amrit he became Guru Gobind Singh.

At the time of the Amrit, Guru Gobind Singh directed that all males should take the name *Singh* after their first name. *Singh* means lion and indicates one who is in control of his animal nature and lives as the regal lion of his own consciousness in the fearless glory of the One God. He told all women to take the name *Kaur* after their first name. *Kaur* means princess and indicates a lady who is the living image of the Grace of God.

His final act, however, was even more extraordinary. All the Gurus before him had named their successor prior to the time of their death and in a simple ceremony, set the succeeding Guru upon the dais. For centuries the Guru had always been identified in the embodiment of a man. Yet Guru Gobind Singh, before his death, installed the *Adi Granth* of Guru Arjun, modified by him with the addition of the writings of his father, Guru Tegh Bahadur, the ninth Guru, as the *Siri Guru Granth Sahib*. He declared that after him the living Guru would be embodied in the Word as found in the *Siri Guru Granth Sahib*. Never again would man bow to man. For in the coming age man would only bow to the Word, as he had done in the Beginning. Guru Gobind Singh's act of installing the *Siri Guru Granth Sahib* as the living Guru marked a turning point in the evolution of the consciousness of Mankind.

In his own writings, Guru Gobind Singh described his previous incarnation. At that time he was a great rishi in the Himalayas, known as Rishi Dusht Dhaman. Now God wanted Rishi Dusht Dhaman to take the incarnation as the last Sikh Guru and turn people away from the cults of personality, bringing mankind to bow before the Word, as Man had done in the Beginning.

After Guru Gobind Singh, the Sikhs entered into a dark and bloody period marked by gruesome combat. They were heavily persecuted by the Moguls and thousands of Sikhs were slaughtered. For years they lived in the forests or in the saddle, fighting to survive. In two devastating massacres, thousands of women, children, and old men were brutally butchered. There was a price on the head of every Sikh. Still they persevered.

By the beginning of the 19th century, the Sikhs were reestablishing themselves as a community in northern India. Soon the Punjab came under the domain of Maharaja Ranjit Singh, the Lion of the Punjab. It was Maharaja Ranjit Singh who covered the Harimander Sahib with gold and marble, causing it to be known later as the Golden Temple. Under Maharaja Ranjit Singh, the Sikh culture flourished through art, music, and literature. Even the advance of the British occupation of India did not penetrate the Punjab under Maharaj Ranjit Singh. By the middle of the 19th century, however, all of India had come under the rule of the British, and India was changed forever.

The Sikhs, though, prospered under the British Raj and proved to be capable administrators as well as warriors. The British put great trust in the Sikhs who distinguished themselves through their trustworthiness, dependability, and valor. The Sikh Regiment of the Indian Army became one of the most decorated regiments in the world. Later, as India inched her way toward independence from the British, it was the

Sikhs who fought the hardest, making heavy sacrifices for a free and democratic India.

From the time of Guru Nanak until the turn of the 20th century, the Sikh religion was essentially confined to the provinces of northern India. With the colonial expansion of the British and India's subsequent independence (resulting in the loss of a large portion of the Punjab to Pakistan), Sikhs immigrated to nearly every country of the world. In the early 20th century a revitalized spirit was growing among the Sikhs and as they spread across the world, they established gurdwaras in their new homelands.

The latter part of the 20th century was a time of sweeping changes in the world. In the United States, the Great Society was being shaken to its foundation by the war in Viet Nam, the Civil Rights Movement, and the growing counterculture. Hippies, yippies, flower children, and radicals all fanned the flames under the cauldron of America, and it was boiling over. Nineteen sixty-nine was the year of Woodstock. It was the year that Yogi Bhajan came to America and began to teach. It was the 500th anniversary of the birth of Guru Nanak. The East and the West had met.

The long, slow sunrise in the West began with Yogi Bhajan in 1969. This book tells the story of one humble man and many young people who shared a dream and who have sacrificed to make that dream a reality. The Sikhs of the West have not had to face trial by *mortal* combat, but they have had to face trial by *moral* combat.

This tale does not tell it all. History is the story of people, and each person who has walked this path has faced his own challenges and tests. In many cases those stories remain untold. This book does tell the story of the whole, however, and tells it beautifully. Simply, we were hippies or students, young and restless. By the Grace of God we had the chance to be part of history. This book is really the tale of how far the hand of the Guru can reach and how, when the wheel of destiny turns, all things fall into place.

It could correctly be said that Sikh Dharma has taken root in the West because it was the Will of God and those who had the destiny to be part of it have played their roles. This book tells the story of grit and commitment and how, when lesser things are sacrificed for greater things, the greatest things happen.

Singh Sahib Gurutej Singh Khalsa

Chapter One

Khalsa is Born in the West
1969-1971

A story is told that once when Guru Gobind Singh and his Sikhs were traveling near the village of Soheva, he came across a grove of jand *trees. Here they decided to make their camp. When they were set up, the Guru asked his soldiers to find a* peepal *tree—a fig tree. His men protested that the climate was too dry, and that the peepal tree would only grow in areas of sufficient water. Still, the Guru insisted they go and look. After the men had searched without success, one Sikh climbed the tallest of the jand trees and surveyed the area. There was not a peepal tree in sight. However, when he climbed down, wedged and protected in the trunk of that same tall jand tree, he discovered the small, white sapling of a young peepal tree. The Guru said, "This tender sapling will grow into a mighty tree. When it overshadows this giant jand tree, that is the time when my Khalsa will spread to the four corners of the world. Then the spirit of the Khalsa which I have enshrined under the command of the Creator shall set up a world society which will last for five thousand years. That Divine society will enjoy peace and affluence."*

Chapter One

The Miracle of Guru Ram Das

The early morning light streaks bands of pink and red into the sky above the beautiful Golden Temple of Amritsar, and the cool air carries the celestial music of Gurbani Kirtan over the waters of the holy tank of Guru Ram Das. The glow of dawn radiates from the gold and marble of Harimandir Sahib as people leave their early morning prayers, walking along the marble parkarma to begin their day. This is the same as it has been for hundreds of years in the old city of Amritsar, but today there is something remarkably different. In the crowd you will see a large group of bright, young, western children in the traditional white dress of the Sikhs, leaving their morning meditation for another day of school. Coming to study in India from America, Canada, South America, and Europe, these are the children of Sikh Dharma of the Western Hemisphere. They are the miracle of Guru Ram Das and the beginning of the fulfillment of Guru Gobind Singh's prophesy: the birth of the Khalsa in the West.

> *Dhan dhan Raam Daas Gur, jin siriaa tinai saavaria*
> *Pooree hoe karaamaat aap sirjanhaarai dhaaria*
>
> *Blessed, blessed is Guru Ram Das, the Lord who created you alone has decorated you. Perfect is Your miracle. The Creator Himself as installed You upon the throne.*
> Siri Guru Granth Sahib pg. 968

Guru Ram Das began his life as Jetha, a poor orphan boy who sold wheatberries on the street to feed himself. That he could rise in spiritual status to become the sovereign leader of the Sikhs is the miracle that the *Siri Guru Granth Sahib* tells us about. So also is it a miracle of Guru Ram Das that Sikh Dharma could find root and grow strong in the countries of the West, far from the green fields of the Punjab. It has grown not through ancestry, but through the commitment of those souls who chose to walk on the path of Nanak.

The birth of Sikh Dharma in the West began in the United States of America in 1969. This was a time of great change and turmoil in the western world. Torn by rapidly changing personal, political, and economic standards, America was in the middle of a cultural revolution that rocked the established social order. The young people of the West were burning with the longing to evolve and develop in the realms of the spirit and soul. Many rejected the values and traditions of their families and communities and began a journey of consciousness to seek a higher meaning in life. Their hair grew long, their idealism soared, and an entire generation searched for purpose and inspiration, sometimes wandering without direction across the highways of America.

"There was never a general proclamation in the United States of America that young people should now begin to grow their hair, yet there was a period of history when the planet Uranus began its progression from the West toward the East. At that time, on the 5th of January, 1969, the people of the West began to change their style of life, and they began to search for true spiritual values. They began to live in the form which God had given them. They had no right direction at that time, so many became sidetracked into drugs and into other less spiritually enlightening activities. But some were destined to receive the Word of Truth, and God did send His message and sent Yogi Bhajan to carry that message to the youth of America."[1]

It was into this milieu that Siri Singh Sahib Bhai Sahib Harbhajan Singh Khalsa Yogiji first arrived in Los Angeles in late December, 1968.

The Guru's Messenger

He was born Harbhajan Singh Puri on August 26, 1929, in the village of Kot Harkarn, Tehsil Wazirabad, in the district of Gujaranwala, a part of the Punjab that is now Pakistan. The future leader of Sikh Dharma of the Western Hemisphere had many teachers throughout his life as his inquisitive mind and thirst for knowledge led him onwards in his spiritual pursuits. His first teacher was his saintly grandfather, Bhai Fateh Singh, who guided him as a young boy. Together they would walk and discuss the subtle nature of the divine and the soul, exploring the depth and expression of the spirit.

Each morning they would rise early, and together they would sit and recite the morning prayers of the Sikhs. First his grandfather would recite his banis and the young Harbhajan Singh would listen, then Bhai Fateh Singh would listen as his grandson prayed in the cool air of the Amrit Vela, that time of stillness in the very early morning before the rising of the sun.

Once he asked his grandfather: "Grandpa, why do you bow so long and deep during your prayer time?" He laughed, and brought Harbhajan to stand in front of a mirror.

"Grandson, how do I look to you?"

Young Harbhajan said, "Grandpa, you look very great, you look very holy and really look like a saint!"

Again, he laughed warmly and said, "You, in your innocence, know me as nothing but a saint. It is only by God's grace that I was born into a family where it is traditional to retain a saintly appearance. I have to pray and meditate, but that is my own responsibility. Perhaps if I were born under a different longitude and latitude, a different *tantra*, I would have been born in a family where this saintly appearance would have been the last result. You know, neither do I have to walk with saffron robes, nor do I have to go and sit in a graveyard. I can sit in my own house, on my own estate surrounded by my family, and still I look saintly. With an attitude of gratitude for this blessing of birth, I always bow."

When he was still very young, Harbhajan Singh studied with a powerful and saintly teacher, Sant Hazara Singh. A vibrant leader and sage, Sant Hazara Singh could recite the entire *Siri Guru Granth Sahib* by heart, and was deeply immersed into the meaning and concept of the Guru's words. He was an accomplished horseman and martial artist, a master of Kundalini Yoga, and the Mahan Tantric of his time. He was also a very strict disciplinarian and an exacting teacher. By the grace of God and Guru, at the age of 16½ Harbhajan Singh mastered Kundalini Yoga, a tool that would serve to uplift and enkindle the hearts of the people of the western world.

It was Yogi Bhajan's destiny to be a leader and a teacher throughout the 39 years he lived in India. As recalled by Sardar Shamsher Singh, PhD, who spent time with him during his college years and early days in New Delhi: "As I look back to the college days, I think of him as a sentinel who felt compelled from within to maintain order around himself. I think of him as a reformer who took upon himself the task of defining and defending social values. I think of him as a sportsman who loved and enjoyed teamwork. I also think of him as a soldier who never lost, and as a philosopher trying to fathom the unknown."[2]

Yogi Bhajan spent a total of 18 years in the service of the Indian Government. Throughout this time, he earned a reputation of courage under fire and absolute integrity in all matters. Yogi Bhajan was a formidable figure: a leader, a teacher, a master of many yogic disciplines, and a champion of Sikh issues. He worked enthusiastically and fought courageously for the cause of the Sikh community.

Although he was renowned as a knowledgeable and powerful yogi, he yearned for a deeper, personal understanding and experience of God. In 1960 Yogi Bhajan chose a government posting in the holy City of Amritsar, and in humility and devotion he rose in the very early morning and washed the floors of the Harimandir Sahib, the Golden Temple, each day for four and one-half years. "When I qualified and realized and experienced myself as a yogi, and when the world around me acknowledged me as a yogi, even then I needed the Guru's Grace. I had to mop the floors of the Harimandir for a long time to clean my own slate."[3]

By cleaning the floors of his beloved Guru's House, he grew in love and dedication to Guru Ram Das. Through this deep personal connection, he discovered that the way to God was through humility and the fulfillment he was seeking could be found only through selfless service.

"What I am today didn't just happen right away. It took me four and one-half years of washing the marble floors of the Golden Temple through a voluntary effort, through the grace of God and Guru. It was the act of mopping the floors of the Golden Temple which mopped all of the dirt out of me. It was nothing else. I could not shine without that rub. The cub shall never rise to the maturity of radiance as a full lion without rubbing the marble floors of the Golden Temple. It is my experience, and I would like to share it with you. The Harimandir Sahib is the nucleus of a spiritually powerful center where the heavens and earth meet to bring harmony. It is not only in India. The Golden Temple is at two places, not just at one place. One is located in the heart of the seeker, the Sikh, and the other is on the Earth in the City of Amritsar."[4]

His decision to leave his lucrative and prestigious job and travel to the West surprised his associates and friends. Always in tune with the higher nature of life, Yogi Bhajan was responding to an inner call, a sense of destiny that others could not perceive. He knew that his mission was to go out and serve the people of the West, bringing to them the joy and wisdom of the Sikh teachings. In the fall of 1968, he traveled to Canada and then to the United States, leaving his wife and three children in India until the time when he could have them join him.

The Sacred Science of Kundalini Yoga

When Yogi Bhajan arrived in America, the distress and confusion he saw in the youth deeply disturbed him. With their long hair and new idealism, they had challenged society and posed questions of consciousness that demanded answers. But these people with great potential and inner spirituality were without direction, searching for answers that were not forthcoming. The youth of America was standing at a crossroads of culture and time, not knowing which way to turn.

Yogi Bhajan delivered his first lecture in Los Angeles on January 5, 1969, and his words dramatically awakened the young people who heard him. He brought them an inspiring message of hope and truth. He said, "Each person must deeply understand why he is a human being and what it means to be a human being. There is a lot of talk and philosophy about this, but remember that intellectual knowledge does not hold and sustain you. Knowledge only becomes real wisdom when you ***experience*** it with your own heart and your own Being. Once you have seen the joy of being a Human Being and have enjoyed the beauty of it, this is an experience of wisdom. **You have a right to be Healthy. You have a right to be Happy. You have a right to be Holy. It is your birthright!"**

Yogi Bhajan knew that the science of Kundalini Yoga gave the technology of mind, spirit, and body that could bring direction and awareness to these young seekers of truth. "Kundalini Yoga is the yoga of awareness. Awareness is a finite relationship with infinity. It is the active interaction of you as a finite individual identity with you as an infinite potential identity. This dormant energy of awareness is in you. Kundalini Yoga is the supreme technology to awaken that awareness and take you into your original self."

The science of Kundalini Yoga had been taught secretly for centuries in India. Shrouded in mystery and myth, it remains one of the most secret of the yogic traditions today. Prior to the advent of Yogi Bhajan's classes in America, it was never taught openly or to novice students. In India, the student had to spend many years preparing to receive this knowledge proving his humility, worthiness, and loyalty. However, Yogi Bhajan recognized that this powerful science could propel those young minds, disenchanted by a meaningless society, into a fulfilling life of grace and consciousness.

Nothing short of Kundalini Yoga could repair the nerves and open the hearts of those people longing to know themselves, to know God, and to achieve their highest potential. It was then that he decided to stay in Los Angeles, and began teaching the science he had mastered in India when only 16½ years old. In a bold step of destiny, he broke the ancient traditions and restrictions and taught Kundalini Yoga to all who came to his classes.

One of the first things Yogi Bhajan taught his students was, **"There is no liberation without labor and there is no freedom which is free."** Classes were long and strenuous, challenging the spirit and endurance of the teenagers who came. He guided and encouraged them through these first steps of consciousness with good humor and infinite patience. Through the process of cleansing their bodies and focusing their minds, their efforts attuned them to the wisdom and spirit within themselves.

"Kundalini Yoga teaches you the techniques and awareness to stay healthy. You gain a strong immune system, glandular and nervous systems. This foundation gives you energy and lets you deal with the mental and spiritual facets of your life. Kundalini Yoga develops your relationship to your mental potential. You learn to use the clarity of the neutral, intuitive, comprehensive mind. You sharpen the intellect, and you act with grace and commitment from your heart."[5]

Many beautiful young people came to learn Kundalini Yoga from Yogi Bhajan and almost immediately their lives began to change. Some of the students were making a transition away from drug use, which was rampant in the turbulent days of the 60s, toward the life of a clean-living yogi. Their lives became charged with a new meaning and a new purpose. They were so enchanted with the path of spiritual awakening that they wholeheartedly pursued Kundalini Yoga and the technology he taught with boundless energy. It soon became the focal point of their activities, and every aspect of their life began to change.

In order to be exalted in the spirit, Yogi Bhajan taught that you had to respect and nourish the physical body. He explained to his students the negative effects of eating meat, drinking alcohol, and smoking cigarettes in a very scientific language that made sense to them. Soon they started eating wholesome, healthy foods, shedding some of their destructive habits. This alone changed and improved the lives of many, many people. He introduced a delicious drink he called "Yogi Tea," a healthy blend of spices, milk, and honey, which took the place of coffee and other stimulant drinks. The delightful smell of Yogi Tea brewing became a familiar pleasure.

Standing tall and dignified with a jet black beard and crisply wrapped turban, Yogi Bhajan was a unique and outstanding individual. His piercing eyes danced with intensity, mystery, and mastery, seeing beyond the physical realities of existence into the innate and subtle nature of each student's heart. He was a wellspring of knowledge about every aspect of life. Through classes, endless discussion, and humbly sharing his life with them, Yogi Bhajan guided his students through the process of self-discovery with patience and tolerance. Powerful yet gentle, he was a master of life, continually broadening their view of reality. All agreed that they had never met anyone like him.

News of this wise teacher in Los Angeles spread, and more and more students came to learn from him. He taught Kundalini Yoga classes at 10:00 AM and 6:30 PM in the showroom of an antique store owned by Jules Buccieri, at the corner of Melrose and Robertson. Every day the students would faithfully move the furniture aside to make space for the yoga class, and move it back when the class was over. Within a few weeks it was obvious they needed a more permanent location. So, with mops, brooms, paint, and devotion they transformed the garage behind the antique shop into a beautiful place of spirituality. The walls were hung with silk, fresh flowers decorated the simple altar, and incense filled the room. They hung a wooden sign over the door carving into it the words, "Guru Ram Das Ashram."

Within a few months hundreds of people were attending classes and the 3HO Foundation was born—the Healthy, Happy, Holy Organization. His students affectionately called him "Yogiji," and a bond of spiritual commitment grew among the people who came to his inspiring and challenging classes.

Opening the Guru's Door

The vision that brought Yogi Bhajan to the West was a deep faith that the Sikh technology was a vital key to the future of humanity. For the most part, people were not looking for a new religion when they came to his Kundalini Yoga classes. But as their lives began to change and their hearts and minds were opened, they yearned to experience the spiritual nature of life. Yogi Bhajan told many captivating stories about the Sikh Gurus and the tests and challenges they championed through courage and faith. His students were drawn to the graceful, powerful, and dignified lifestyle of the Sikhs.

"[Yogi Bhajan] is the first glorious son of Guru Gobind Singh who approached these western youth. He met them, cared for them, loved them, and brought them to the feet of his Guru. He instructed them in the fundamentals of the Sikh faith and bade them to earn their living by honest labor, to meditate on God's Name, and to share their earnings with the needy and poor. Through his soul-stirring lectures, they were awakened into a new life. And it is Guru's wonder that he transformed them from hippies to yoga students, and from yoga students to Sikhs and from Sikhs to Khalsa."[6]

In the manner of the Sikh tradition, Yogi Bhajan taught his students to rise early to meditate each day, a practice known as *sadhana*. Although the word *sadhana* simply means "spiritual practice," for a Sikh it begins by rising at 3:00 AM and taking a very cold shower. In the chilly predawn hours, people came to Guru Ram Das Ashram warmly wrapped in their meditation blankets, carrying their mats to sit on. With a deep sincerity and a lightness of soul, they came together to chant according to the Sikh teachings:

Gur sat gur kaa jo sikh akhaae, So bhalake uth Harnaam dhiaavai
Udam kare bhalake parbhaatee, Ishnaan kare Amritsar naavai
Upades Guru Har Har jap jaapai, Sabh kilavikh paap dokh leh jaavai
Fir charai divas gurbaanee gaavai, Behediaa uthadiaa Harnam
dhiaavai

One who calls himself a Sikh of the True Guru shall rise in the early
morning hours and meditate on God's Name. Upon arising, he is to
bathe and cleanse himself in the Nectar Tank. Following the
instructions of the Guru, he is to chant the Name of the Lord. All
sins, misdeeds, and negativity shall be erased. Then, at the rising of
the sun, he is to sing Gurbani, whether sitting or standing, he is to
meditate on God's Name.

Guru Ram Das Ji
Siri Guru Granth Sahib, pg. 305

In every class and lecture, Yogi Bhajan emphasized the importance of a daily morning sadhana. "Somebody asked me what sadhana does. I said, 'Nothing.' He said, 'Well, it must be doing something. You all the time say, 'sadhana, sadhana, sadhana.' I said, 'Sadhana is nothing but where a disciplined one, the love or lover talks to the One.' Sadhana is where you clean your own mind. Sadhana is where one prepares for the day to become kind and compassionate for everyone, including your enemies. Desperation, depression, and a feeling of destitution come only to those who have no discipline or sadhana. A house which is not cleaned looks dirty, and the mind which is not cleansed stinks as well. Sadhana is self-cleaning. When you want to be blissful and bountiful, you have to have a clear mind, a mind through which your spirit and your soul can shine."[7]

For many of these young people, there was a subliminal familiarity with the Sikh traditions and lifestyle. For the people who had been drawn to Yogi Bhajan and the Sikh teachings, there was often a feeling of "coming home," a deep sense of "remembering," and they began to come together to live as a community of spiritual people. Some people came, benefited from the yoga classes, and moved on to other aspects of their life, bringing with them the lessons learned from the Sikh technology. All were welcomed in whatever large or small way they chose to participate, and "Sat Nam" could be heard echoing up and down Melrose Avenue.

On Sunday nights, students would stay after yoga class to share music, food, and the company of each other. People played guitars and sang, composing many beautiful songs about God and their awakening to a spiritual life. The music served to bond and uplift the fledgling Sikhs, and they poured their hearts out into these devotional songs. In a world with too many questions and not enough answers, Sunday night kirtan was a chance to relax with kindred souls and rejoice with people of high spirits and reverent idealism. For many people, it was the high point of their week.

One day some of his students brought to class a song written by a rock and roll group, The Incredible String Band. It was a simple tune of love and innocence that captured the joy of the times. Yogi Bhajan ended every class with this song, as he still does today: *"May the long time sun shine upon you, all love surround you, and the pure light within you, guide your way on."*

Music was the primary channel of expression for the 3HO students, for words alone could not convey the passion and excitement they felt during this time of personal growth and transformation. Even at this early juncture, Yogi Bhajan knew that they were the beginning of a strong Khalsa Nation and, as with the Sikhs of Guru Nanak's time, music would play an essential role. He wholeheartedly encouraged and participated in the composition of these inspiring songs. He often said, **"God respects me when I work, but he loves me when I sing!"**

The bond of spiritual identity grew strong between Yogi Bhajan and his students. As was natural, they developed a sincere dedication to this man who had to come to play such an important role in their lives. Continuously, Yogi Bhajan said, "Don't love me, because this is not of my doing. It is all the miracle of Guru Ram Das, so love Him from whom this wisdom flows. I am just a postman delivering the message to you, and you in turn should share it with others."

He taught them that a Sikh would bow to no man, and that they should worship only the One Creator of all. He made it very clear to the many students who came to learn from him that he was not, and could not be, their guru. He had come to America to bring the message of Guru Nanak and to share with the people of the West the freedom and joy of coming to the feet of Guru Ram Das.

When this question was posed to him by a student, his reply was consistent and clear: "I am a man. I cannot be your guru, and I do not want the guru-trip. It doesn't suit me. My relationship with you is very simple. I feel that God has blessed me to have some knowledge, and if I can share with my brothers and sisters in faith, and they can enjoy the same ecstasy of consciousness, then we all can enjoy the same joy. I have mopped the floor of the Golden Temple, and I have found the richest riches in my soul. That is why I say, **'Love a man of God and be a man of God, but only worship the One God.'** You shall not bow to anyone other than God, even if you are cut limb by limb, because no man can be a slave to another man. I am no one's guru. I am just a useless pipe, but a good plumber picked me up, and now I quench the thirst of those whose souls are thirsty. I say, 'Hail! Hail! Hail to Guru Ram Das, who picked up this meanest of the men and made him a very meaningful person.'"[8]

Developing a Spiritual Identity

In a little over one year's time, the unrestrained nature of the young people who were coming to yoga classes was beginning to refine into the purity of Khalsa. One of the first things Yogi Bhajan taught his students was to dress all in white as an outward symbol and inner reminder of the purity and consciousness to which they aspired. He taught that wearing white expands the aura, giving the student greater strength in his personal electromagnetic field.

"You are not just this body. Your energy is in your aura and your aura extends nine feet from your skin. There are two things which can increase the size of the aura: white clothes and cotton cloth. When you wear white, cotton clothing from top to bottom, you can increase your aura up to three times. This is under all circumstances, even if you are at your lowest ebb. That's the law of the universe."[9]

Wearing white clothes made each person very conscious of their actions and movements in order to stay clean throughout the day. It also served an important role in creating a sense of identity and unity among the students of Guru Ram Das Ashram.

Slowly, all that wild, long hair became combed and clean, and students started wearing turbans as their Sikh brothers did in India. For both men and women, the beautiful, white turban was a bold declaration of spiritual values and identity.

As part of the transformation these young people were undergoing, many took on spiritual names, leaving their birth names and confirming their new spiritual identity. By taking the last name "Singh" or "Kaur" they committed themselves to walking the path of Nanak, as "seekers of Truth."

"'A rose by any other name would smell as sweet,' or would it? We know the name of a thing is not the thing itself, but the vibration of the name, if it is based on higher awareness, can put you in tune with the thing itself. By the grace of God, Yogi Bhajan has seen fit to bestow upon many of us new names, spiritual names—names that establish a vibration for us to grow into, to expand into, to relate to in consciousness and in being. Never before in the history of America have there been so many 'Singhs' and 'Kaurs' and we are experiencing the psychological and emotional changes that new names stimulate, not only in ourselves but in others. With a new name, we are no longer limited and forced to counteract the vibrations of preconceived ideas about us in other people's minds which are always summoned up by the repetition of the old name. A new name is a new birth."[10]

The Grace of God Movement of America

As Yogi Bhajan continued to deal with the problems of the western culture, he was deeply disturbed by the situation of women in American society. In such a technologically advanced country, he was appalled that women were used and abused as sex symbols. He knew that when women are denied dignity, grace, and their rightful status in society, generation after generation of children will suffer. He taught, **"When a man falls, an individual falls. But when a woman falls, an entire generation is lost."**

On September 22, 1970, in San Francisco, he began a campaign for the upliftment of the women of the western world. He told them, "You are the grace of the individual, you are the grace of the town, you are the grace of the nation, you are the grace of the world. The world starts with you, and it ends with you. Therefore, you should never be cheap. When you cannot handle what you are, you become cheap. The crown of grace, divinity, and dignity should be on your head, and it should not create a headache for you. Therefore, you have to be trained. You have to train your emotions, you have to train yourself, and you have to go one way. There is one way to One God for a woman: selfless, dignified, and graceful behavior. Dignity and divinity are your birthright."

He taught a special mediation to the women that established and confirmed their grace and radiance. With a relaxed and meditative mind, they chanted, "I am the Grace of God." That night The Grace of God Movement was born, and it became the strength and dignity of an entire generation of women. With candles in hand, his students marched in procession through Northbeach, the red-light district of San Francisco, past the nude bars and the porno theaters, chanting "We are the Grace of God." The city, with its nightlife in full swing, looked on in wonder and amazement.

"I am not doing anything new in this country; after all, you do celebrate Mother's Day. I am just telling women that 'You are the Grace of God.' All I am trying to do is remind the mother of her responsibilities and telling the men that they are born of the woman. If there is no respect for the woman, there shall be no peace on this earth. This is what I believe, I will stand by it, and this is what I am going to preach.

"I have seen through your lifestyle. How can a man, born out of a woman, become so shameless that he allows women to give service in a restaurant totally naked? How can that happen in such a civilized country? Well, that exists and I know it does. The signs are advertising it just two blocks from where I live. This big hypocrisy in which you and I are participating is very evident. But there is a method to face this untruth, and I am adopting this method: to raise the consciousness of the people, to make them aware, and to make them realize the Truth in mankind." [11]

Coming to the Guru's Feet

On Baisakhi Day, 1970, two young students decided they wanted to "officially" become Sikhs and requested that Yogiji initiate them. At that time and many times since, he has replied, "My birth and my life and my end are meant to serve, to console, to inspire, to share the sufferings and to take the suffering, and that is my happiness. I firmly, honestly and truthfully feel that I am much, much, and very much lower than the dust under the feet of those who have uttered 'Sat Nam' once, and that too by mistake. You remember when I came to the United States? Up to this day, I have not initiated any single person. How can I initiate any man into a spiritual way of life when he himself is born out of the Infinite Soul?" [12]

Yogi Bhajan instructed these young men to go to the *Siri Guru Granth Sahib*, who is the only Guru of any Sikh. Since the young American Sikhs did not yet have the *Siri Guru Granth Sahib* available to them, they went to the Sikh Study Circle of Los Angeles, a prominent Sikh Gurdwara in the area. Charged with spiritual energy and vision, they presented themselves before the *Siri Guru Granth Sahib* dressed in white and with beautiful white turbans. When they announced their intentions to the sangat, the Gurdwara management did not know what to do with them! They had never seen someone who was not of Indian origin wanting to become a Sikh. One of them phoned Guru Ram Das Ashram to ask Yogi Bhajan what he thought they should do. He advised them that all they had to do was give these young men to the *Siri Guru Granth Sahib.* That was all.

A simple ceremony was improvised on the spot. Two men from the congregation offered their own karas so that the new Sikhs could have them to wear. These two young men with sparkling eyes and pure hearts were presented by the Gurdwara President to the sangat. In the weeks that followed, many more yoga students took Sikh vows. For the first time in history, people of the western world were adopting the form and teachings of the Sikh Gurus, bowing their head to the *Siri Guru Granth Sahib.*

In Los Angeles, Yogi Bhajan's students began attending Sunday morning Gurdwara services at the Sikh Study Circle with him. Because of their love of devotional music, several students learned to sing Gurbani Kirtan. Even though Gurmukhi script was difficult for the American Sikhs to learn, they were longing to understand the prayers and mantras they were reciting daily. Taking translations of the Sikh daily prayers, Sardarni Premka Kaur was absorbed for weeks writing them in poetic verse that could be easily understood by western Sikhs. The resulting book, *Peace Lagoon,* contained translations of the daily prayers of the Sikhs, known as the *banis,* as well as selections from the *Sukhmani Sahib,* the *Lavan*—the wedding prayer of the Sikhs, and the *Sidha Gosht* of Guru Nanak. In the summer of 1971, *Peace Lagoon* was published by the Brotherhood of Life Bookstore in Albuquerque, New Mexico. It is still today the primary translation used by people new to the Sikh faith in the West.

Even so, this was not enough to quench the inexhaustible desire of the new western sangat to learn the teachings of the Sikh Gurus. They were yearning to experience this knowledge firsthand, directly from the source. In August of 1971, Yogi Bhajan was able to obtain copies of the English translation of the *Siri Guru Granth Sahib* by Manmohan Singh and distributed them. A wave of breathless excitement rippled through Sikh Dharma as the Guru was lovingly installed in the Guru Ram Das Ashrams.

Yogi Bhajan deeply ingrained the love and devotion for the *Siri Guru Granth Sahib* in the hearts of the new Sikhs. "The *Siri Guru Granth Sahib* is not a book, my friend. It is not a paper, my friend. It is not a Gurmukhi, my friend. It is not only Gurbani, my friend. It is Guru, my friend, and it is nothing but that. The Word of the Guru *is* a Guru in life, in communication, in vibration. This is the miracle of the rebirth of the Khalsa, 'the pure ones,' which even the ordinary man can understand, but only the faithful can practice. What a great moment it is on this day that we are reciting these words, as Guru Nanak got hold of this idea and left it to Guru Arjan to compile the words of the Guru's and the men who were immersed in God-consciousness, so that we who are to follow can exactly recite and train ourselves in that state of ecstasy of consciousness."[13]

The India Yatra of 1970

After being away from India for nearly two years, in December of 1970 Yogi Bhajan returned to the country of his birth with a group of 84 students. When the Americans visited the Golden Temple at Amritsar, they touched the roots from which they had grown. For the first time the new western Sikhs were bathed in the golden light reflecting from the walls of the Harimandir Sahib, absorbing them in the love of Guru Ram Das.

Bowing their heads in the Harimandir Sahib was a transformational experience for them, locking the destiny of Sikh Dharma in the West. Never before had they experienced anything equal to the majesty and spiritual eminence of the House of Guru Ram Das. The power of that experience culminated years of searching and longing. They realized that it was to Guru Ram Das that they truly belonged. They had come home at last.

So moved were they by this first experience at the Harimandir Sahib that many of the young Sikhs asked to receive the sacred Amrit, to be initiated into the fellowship of the Khalsa. They reverently prepared themselves, and in the pre-dawn hours they walked with Yogiji around the marble parkarma to the door of the Akal Takhat. Here he stopped and with a gentle hand on their shoulder, he sent them up the stairs alone, telling them: "I have brought you to the Guru's feet, and now my job is done. The rest of the distance you must walk alone."

After giving Amrit, the Jathedar of the Akal Takhat gave turbans to the young Americans, welcoming them with an open heart into the order of the Khalsa. The Jathedar saw with certainty that the winds of change were blowing for the Sikhs of the world! For the first time in history, men and women born in the West were standing before the *Siri Guru Granth Sahib* as sons and daughters of Guru Gobind Singh.

They traveled in buses from gurdwara to gurdwara, meeting the sangat and getting their first exposure to the Indian culture. The people in India had heard news of this missionary from the West, and thousands of people packed the gurdwaras to see the western, white-clad Sikhs. The group did not yet have much knowledge of Sikh Dharma, but they had love of Guru in their hearts, and they sang spirited tunes of *Ek Ong Kar Sat Nam Siri Wahe Guru* and *Bhaja Mana Mayray Hari Ka Naam* for the congregations. The western jatha made a deep impression on the people of Punjab, and were received with great love and acceptance.

They visited many powerful and respected spiritual people during their tour of India. It happened that early in the tour, a Sant wanted the American Sikhs to come and accept him as their living guru. Yogiji refused, stating that his Guru was Guru Ram Das, and it was to the feet of Guru Ram Das that these Americans were coming. As

Yogi Bhajan tells it, "A very saintly man challenged me that if Guru Ram Das is really my Guru, then he must have given me a Guru Mantra. I told him that every Sikh has the Guru Mantra and that is *Wahe Guru*. But he was challenging me that if Guru Ram Das was my personal Guru, then he should be in a position to give me His mantra.

"So I said, 'Okay, I will meditate and I'll see. If Guru Ram Das loves me, he may appear; if not, I can't say.' So the next day I was chanting *Wahe Guru, Wahe Guru, Wahe Guru,* in the way, the tone, the method, the technology with which the Guru Mantra is to be chanted. After a little while I was surprised to find that there was a pure light in that room and then a human being was sitting there in the very visible form of Guru Ram Das.

"And thus spoke the great Guru: 'At this time you need the protection of a mantra. The people who are following you are not yet ripe. Chant this: *Guru Guru Wahe Guru, Guru Ram Das Guru.* You do not want to claim anything as your own achievement, and you don't want to take the blame either. Let the claim be mine, and let me also take the blame. Now say this mantra.' And I started saying it slowly, hesitantly, and I liked it.

"Then I ran and told that man that I had actually seen Guru Ram Das in a very beautiful light and form. He got very annoyed because he thought he could prove that I have to come to him as my guru. He told me that *he* would show me the truth. After that they did make plans and attempts to kill me and to do other things to us, but that mantra did protect us throughout the entire ordeal."[14]

The western jatha soon began chanting and singing this new mantra day and night, and an envelope of joy and protection surrounded the group. As never before they felt loved and sheltered by the hand of Guru Ram Das.

In New Delhi, they set up tents and camped in a mango grove outside the city. Here they received guests and traveled to gurdwaras in the vicinity. Things were going well, except that the altar in Yogi Bhajan's meditation room caught fire several days in a row. Although every precaution was taken, somehow the altar would again catch fire. At this time, Yogi Bhajan had another vision that guided the destiny of the group.

"I saw a man on a horse who was less than five feet and six inches, in the perfect body of Guru Gobind Singh, but without a head! There was no head on his body and instead in that place there was a huge flame! So I asked, 'Guru Ji, what is this, there is no head?' And he replied, 'Hard times will come on you. Dharma will spread, but I have to return these seeds which you have brought with you from across the ocean. Follow me and I will carry you safely across, and then we will see what Khalsa will be.'"

When the missionary work being done by Yogi Bhajan in America came to the attention of the Sikh leadership in Amritsar, they were profoundly inspired. A new era for Sikh Dharma was unfolding as the barriers of language, country, and culture were slowly dissolving. "Soon after Yogi Bhajan's arrival he was welcomed by Giani

Mahinder Singh, the Secretary of the S.G.P.C.,[15] who was delighted and amazed to see the students who had been guided to the house of Guru Ram Das, and he immediately appreciated the missionary work that was so effectively being carried on in the West by this one inspired Gursikh. Yogi Bhajan met with other leaders, including Sant Chanan Singh, the President of the S.G.P.C., and Sant Fateh Singh, President of the Shiromani Akali Dal, to discuss his missionary work in the West. It was determined that Yogiji should be honored at the Akal Takhat for his achievements, and that he should be presented with a letter of authority from the S.G.P.C. to establish a Ministry for Sikh Dharma in the Western Hemisphere.

"In the course of the discussion, Sant Fateh Singh indicated that Yogiji should be given a saropa and a Siri Sahib (sword of honor) from the Akal Takhat and that he should be called by the title of 'Singh Sahib.' At that point, Sant Chanan Singh spoke up and said: 'What do you mean? This one Harbhajan Singh will create *many* Singh Sahibs! We are presenting him with a Siri Sahib, so let us call him 'Siri Singh Sahib!'"[16]

On March 3, 1971, in a beautiful ceremony before a huge congregation, the Jathedar of the Akal Takhat presented Yogi Bhajan with a sword of honor, and he was entrusted with the responsibility to establish the Ministry of the Sikhs in the Western Hemisphere. From that day on, Yogi Bhajan came to be known by the respected title of "Siri Singh Sahib." This bold step of destiny by the Sikh leadership in Amritsar laid the foundation for the future growth of Sikh Dharma in the countries of the western world.

Toward the end of the tour, the jatha arrived at the gurdwara in Patiala. As in dozens of other gurdwaras across India, the western jatha sang the few mantras they knew, and the sangat received them with great warmth and enthusiasm. But as they sang, a commotion broke out in the back of the gurdwara. People began pushing and shouting, and angry voices directed at the Siri Singh Sahib could be heard over the kirtan. The men sitting in the sangat enjoying the kirtan became angry with the interlopers, and as they tried to control the situation, a near riot ensued. Suddenly, shots rang out in the gurdwara. Without hesitation, the western Sikhs surrounded the Siri Singh Sahib and pushed him to the ground, lying down on top of him to protect him from the gunfire with their own bodies.

He was deeply touched and humbled by the love and devotion shown to him by the young Sikhs. Here in the country of his birth, where he had lived and served with distinction for 39 years, he had been betrayed by treachery and violence. It was the beautiful new Sikhs who faced death without hesitation to protect him.

The Gift of White Tantric Yoga

When he returned to America, the Siri Singh Sahib accelerated his teaching and travel schedule in order to reach more and more students across the United States and Canada. One morning in the spring of 1971, the Siri Singh Sahib came out early from his morning meditation and announced to his students that an extraordinary thing had happened. The mantle of the "Mahan Tantric" had just been passed to him. No one had ever heard of that before, and they asked him what he meant. The Siri Singh Sahib patiently explained.

In his youth, he had studied with a very powerful and saintly teacher, Sant Hazara Singh, who was the Mahan Tantric of his time. Together with a few other students, Yogi Bhajan went through many tests and acquired vast amounts of spiritual knowledge. Although there were other students who matched Yogi Bhajan's aptitude, he knew that he was the best, and he was sure that when the time came the power of the Mahan Tantric would be given to him. It was because of this pride that when Sant Hazara Singh died, the mastery of the Mahan Tantric was given to another student, Lama Lilan Po of Tibet. He further explained that only one person at a time carried this sacred responsibility, and Lama Lilan Po had just died, passing on the power of the Mahan Tantric to the Siri Singh Sahib.

This event had far-reaching effects on the mission of Sikh Dharma in the West, because White Tantric Yoga is very different from other forms of yoga. During the practice of White Tantric Yoga, the infinite energy of the universe is channeled through the Mahan Tantric to all the participants, cleansing and purifying the subconscious mind and freeing the participants of deep-rooted mental blocks, fears, and anger. This divine technology cannot be practiced without the direct guidance of the Mahan Tantric, because it is through his own consciousness that the negativity and subconscious blocks of the participant's mind are filtered and released.

"During White Tantra the infinite energy of the universe flows through the Mahan Tantric into all of the participants. White Tantric Yoga is no ordinary yoga. It cannot be practiced without the Mahan Tantric present because it takes his mastery over emotions for it to be not only effective but safe. Partners face each other in straight lines while the Mahan Tantric projects his own astral body to encircle them. He thereby extends his own psychoelectromagnetic field to encompass the group aura. During a White Tantric meditation, a lot of subconscious negativity from each participant comes to the surface. In order to release that negativity, the Mahan Tantric filters the negativity through his own consciousness. The participants' aura must change to blue and gold, representing devotion and perfection. White Tantric Yoga needs special circumstances, it has a special teacher, and it yields special results."[17]

With the dynamic energy of White Tantric Yoga, the slow process of purification and refinement of the new yoga students was accelerated. The insight and clarity of mind that normally could take years to achieve through individual meditation could be accomplished in a very short time through White Tantric Yoga.

The first White Tantric Yoga course was held at the Guru Ram Das Ashram on Melrose Avenue. Men and women sat in alternating rows facing each other and performed the kriyas as directed by the Mahan Tantric. The course lasted three days, five to six hours each day. Arms ached and legs hurt from the unaccustomed kriyas, and the ego was mightily tested. All who attended experienced a dramatic transformation within themselves. News of this "new" event spread rapidly through the 3HO Ashrams, and plans were soon made to teach White Tantric Yoga throughout the United States and Canada.

The House of Guru Ram Das

Yogi Bhajan knew if the teachings were to reach all the people destined to hear it, there would need to be many more teachers. He repeatedly told his students, "I have not come to gather disciples. I have come to create teachers ten times greater than I." He had already begun to travel extensively, and Shakti Parwha Kaur covered his classes at the Guru Ram Das Ashram while he was away.

As soon as a yoga student became proficient in the practice of Kundalini Yoga, Yogi Bhajan sent him or her out to different cities in America and all over the world to teach. Early in 1969, an ashram was opened in the San Francisco Bay area. In February, he sent Soorya Kaur to Washington, DC, in advance of his first east coast tour, and she opened the Ahimsa Ashram. Soon, teachers were dispatched to cities all across the United States, Canada, and Europe. 3HO Ashrams were beginning to spring up everywhere. Yogi Bhajan taught, **"First there is individual consciousness, then there is group consciousness and through that there is God Consciousness."**

Most of the ashrams were named after Guru Ram Das and were sanctuaries of peace and consciousness. "Guru Ram Das's house is a house of healing. It is a house of love. It is a house of those who humble themselves. We come here to be blessed, and we are already being blessed when we are walking in this direction. It is the greatest meditation if you walk to the House of Guru Ram Das. And remember, you can expect all miracles in the world, but the greatest miracle that will happen to you will be when you are elevated to the consciousness of the God within you."[18]

It was a brave and difficult thing for these young student-teachers to leave their friends, their fellow students, and their spiritual teacher to start an ashram in a new and strange city. It took courage, faith, and a deep commitment to the mission that they had adopted. "It is the most difficult thing to be a teacher. It is a very heavy situation where I have asked you to become teachers and where the time demands that you become the teachers and leaders of the Age. Remember what I have always taught you: **'If you want to learn a thing, read that, if you want to understand a thing, write that, and if you want to master a thing, teach that.'** You have been handed the banner of 'Sat Nam' to keep it flying, come what may, and there will be many difficulties to test your devotion. So my dear ones, I have not come to this country to create disciples; I have come to create teachers. I am a humble postman, and I am carrying your letters to you, where you can see what is your destiny and what is required. It is up to you to do it, and the time is NOW!"[19]

In Washington, DC, the Ahimsa Ashram was established on Q Street. This ramshackled brownstone was rented for $250 per month and had plenty of room to spare.

Within a matter of months, it was transformed into an ashram, and regular classes and morning sadhana were held there. It quickly grew to become an important center for Sikh Dharma on the east coast, organizing and supporting the ashrams east of the Mississippi that, at times, felt so far removed from the hub of activity in Los Angeles. Strategically located in the Nation's capital, the Ahimsa Ashram was the center for many social activities that involved the Sikhs in the years to follow.

In November of 1971, the students in the ashram in Santa Fe, New Mexico, were told without much notice to move and find someplace else to live. When the Siri Singh Sahib received the call, he told the students to stay together. He told them to go north, and find a place where the sun was shining through the clouds, assuring them that God and Guru would guide them to their destiny.

With faith they drove north to look for a new place for an ashram. The property they found was the only place where the sun was shining that day. It was a humble farmhouse with a barn located on a little over six acres of land. The belabored old buildings dated back to the turn of the century and looked every year of it. There were thousands of old tires stacked in huge mounds and the remains of several wrecked cars that needed to be disposed of. But the group went to work and the property underwent a transformation into the Guru Ram Das Ashram. In the farmhouse, the old apple storeroom became the sadhana room, and the dirt-floored room for vegetable storage became the men's dormitory. Across the hall, the ladies had a room, and the simple kitchen became the heart-center of the ashram where community meals were prepared.

"God guided us to Española, and that is why I have always said that this place never belongs to any person. It belongs to God, because we would never have thought of getting it, and we had no means to get it. It was given to us. Therefore it is a gift of God and Guru."[20]

The Guru Ram Das Ashram on 1620 Preuss Road in Los Angeles was purchased by the Siri Singh Sahib on December 23, 1971, to provide the students and sangat with a permanent base for lectures and classes.[21] A former office building, it required major renovation, remodeling, and landscaping. With loving hands and willing hearts, it was transformed into an oasis of beauty and inspiration. Guru Ram Das Ashram in Los Angeles set the standard for the many other ashrams being established throughout America.

"The ambrosial hours begin the day, and people from all the ashrams in the Los Angeles area come to Guru Ram Das Ashram for morning sadhana. 4:00 AM starts three hours of chanting, exercises, and singing. At 7:00 AM, tea and blanched almonds are served with the closing song, 'May the long time sun shine upon you.' Occasionally we have the added blessing of Yogiji's appearance. Dressed in casual attire, he gives us his unending words of wisdom and inspiration. Everyone would love to stay and listen to Yogiji all day, but he sends us off before it gets too late, with some of his most familiar aphorisms: 'Work is Worship.' 'There is no liberation without labor.' 'Keep Up!'"

"In addition to the regular morning and evening yoga classes taught each day at Guru Ram Das Ashram by many different teachers, Yogiji teaches a beginners class and an advanced class four nights a week. Each class includes a lecture on the science of the soul and an exercise in meditation that gives direct experience of that elevated consciousness."[22]

The Siri Singh Sahib set a rigorous travel schedule to visit and teach at the many ashrams that were now all over the world. Before he went to an ashram, the students spent weeks preparing for the visit. There would be a flurry of activity, cleaning, repairing, and painting each and every thing, and feelings of anticipation ran high. When the Siri Singh Sahib arrived, the first thing he did was inspect the ashram to discover any failing in the cleaning process. Inevitably, he would go directly to the one drawer that hadn't been cleaned, or the closet where the last-minute items had been thrown. Shakti Parwha writes, "On April 14th, the birthday of the Fifth Guru Nanak was celebrated at Guru Arjan Dev Ashram in Brentwood. As Yogiji made his usual tour inspection of the ashram before taking langar, one of the students remarked that everything looked different when seen through the sharp Virgo eyes of Yogi Bhajan! As we all know, Yogiji insists that the ashrams should *always* be immaculately clean and pure, for each ashram is really the House of the Guru."[23]

The concept of the "3HO Family" was the bond that held this fledgling organization together. People lived and worked together in ashrams, rising in the early morning for Sikh prayers, chanting, and the practice of Kundalini Yoga. The commitment to each other they developed was the strength that helped many people continue on the spiritual path. Also, many young people took yoga classes for a short time, benefited by the experience, and moved on to other things. "It is an interesting thing about 'belonging to 3HO,' because there is no way that one can gain membership or lose it. We do not issue membership cards, and Yogi Bhajan does not initiate disciples. Many have come and will come to the Kundalini Yoga classes; they learn what they can assimilate, and then they depart. This is all a part of the divine plan. So, dear ones, many have come to go, and many more will come. To all we send love and prayers and the hope that the seeds of Truth that have been planted will bear fruit."[24]

The Traveling Spiritual Teacher

Yogi Bhajan did not limit his mission to Los Angeles, but traveled extensively to reach the masses across the United States and Canada. There was wide press coverage, interviews on television and in print, and the impact of 3HO was gaining a significant momentum. In 1970 he addressed a large group of young people at the Palm Beach Pop Festival, and in July was invited to speak at the Atlanta Pop Festival. In the spirit of Sikhism, Yogi Bhajan supported and encouraged all people of higher consciousness, regardless of their religious affiliation. He invited many of the spiritual leaders of the time to join him in Atlanta so that people of the various "New Age" spiritual groups would have an opportunity to deliver their messages. This event was lovingly dubbed the "Holy Man Jam." Taking place right on the heels of Woodstock, there were several hundred thousand young music lovers who came to the Atlanta Pop Festival to see the show. Swami Satchidananda, Hari Krishnas, Christians, Buddhists, American Indians, and other religious leaders spoke to the gathering on Yogi Bhajan's invitation. "That Sunday, early in the morning at about 10:00 o'clock, we looked out on the racetrack infield. There must have been about 200,000 completely 'stoned' human beings out there. All these swamis, yogis, Christians, etc., got up and each gave their message, their mantra, or their exercises."[25]

In June of 1970, the 3HO Foundation sponsored its first Summer Solstice Sadhana camp. Starting out in the canyons of the Santa Clara Indian Pueblo in New Mexico, the encampment soon became too large, and they were asked by the local Native Americans to move. Robert Bossier, a man who was to become a good friend of 3HO, graciously offered his nearby land for the remainder of the camp. Fraught with water shortages and unexpected challenges, Yogi Bhajan expounded, **"Keep up and you will be kept up!"** This first 3HO Solstice camp served to unify and coordinate the many students and ashram leaders from both the east and west coasts. Information was exchanged, old friends were reunited, and new students had the chance to meet seekers of consciousness from other parts of America. The annual Summer and Winter Solstice Sadhana still serve this purpose today: to bind, uplift, and unify the world community of Sikh Dharma.

My First Yoga Class

In 1974, I was 21 years old and I decided to go and live in California. A friend gave me the address of the Guru Ram Das Ashram in Los Angeles. She said to go there and I could learn the "Grace of God" meditation.

When I arrived in Los Angeles, I went to the ashram and the receptionist told me to go into the sadhana room to wait for someone to come. The ashram struck me as such a beautiful and peaceful place, a large, open room with no furniture and beautiful paintings hung on the walls. After waiting about an hour, a young woman came in to teach me the meditation. She wore a white kurta with white churidas and a white turban covering her hair. I had never seen anyone like her! She patiently taught me the meditation, but to be honest, the concept of "Grace of God" was beyond what I could understand at the time.

She suggested that I come back for the yoga class that evening, and

I did. I had tried some hatha yoga in New York, and it did not catch my interest. But these exercises were different. Then I had an experience that most people don't have in their first class. We were doing three minutes of "Breath of Fire" in camel pose, and when the time was up and we relaxed out of the position, I had a "kundalini" experience. Suddenly, I was so high, so expanded, I was outside the confinement of my body! I remember thinking, "Wow! So this is why these people do this!" My vision had darkened, my extremities were tingling, and my ears were ringing so loud I could hardly hear. This voice in my head kept getting louder and louder saying, "I'm home. I'm HOME. I'M HOME!"

The class came to an end, and everyone sang "May the long time sun shine upon you...." I was still dazed when I stood up to leave, but as I walked the feeling started to fade. After that, I came to yoga class every night at the Guru Ram Das Ashram.

One night, I came to class and it was unusually full. The room was packed elbow to elbow with all different types of people. There were many people dressed in pure white, some with turbans tied on their heads. They seemed so holy and so special that I felt a little shy so I sat at the back of the room. A tall man in a white turban came in, and I could tell from the pictures I had seen that this man must be Yogi Bhajan. He sat on the teacher's dais, and spoke for almost an hour but I could not understand a single word he said. Others evidently did, because they were scribbling fiercely in notebooks, intent on every word. Finally he led us in a meditation with our eyes closed and our hands cupped like conch shells around our ears. As I was doing the meditation, something made me open my eyes and there he was directly in front of me! He was so close, our noses practically touched, and his eyes were like big, black basketballs staring into mine. After sometime, he put his index finger on my forehead, and I automatically closed my eyes. When I opened them again, he was gone, sitting up on the teacher's platform.

Throughout these past 21 years as a Sikh, I have met many difficult challenges. As I think back to those beginning days, I am renewed with a great strength because I know that Guru Ram Das has blessed me. It was nothing short of a miracle that I came here, and I know, as I knew even then, that it is my destiny and great good fortune to serve the House of Guru Ram Das.

Sat Nirmal Kaur Khalsa
January 20, 1995

The Love of Guru Ram Das

The Siri Singh Sahib told many engaging stories of Guru Ram Das to his yoga students. He talked frequently about Guru Ram Das, not only as the sovereign founder of Amritsar, but also of his service and humility. He related an image of Guru Ram Das as a poor orphan boy who rose to the highest spiritual status, from an unknown street peddler of wheatberries to the throne of the Guru. That such a possibility in life could exist gave inspiration and faith to the many people who came to the House of Guru Ram Das. "By tuning our frequency through devotion and prayer to the attributes of Guru Ram Das, we open our hearts to humility, healing, and service—which is what these times require. The love of Guru Ram Das is a code to release the lock of spirituality in this dark age and to shed the heavy load of spiritual ignorance."[26]

The students of Guru Ram Das Ashram sang and chanted the mantra *Guru Guru Wahe Guru, Guru Ram Das Guru* daily as an exclamation of their love and faith. For the western Sikhs, Guru Ram Das filled the quintessential role of healer, protector, confidant, and intimate companion. Many longed deeply for "a sip and a dip" in the nectar tank of the Golden Temple as their souls were awakened to their spiritual heritage.

As the busy year of 1971 came to a close, there were 57 3HO Ashrams and Kundalini Yoga centers instituted in five countries around the world. Firmly established in the western world, the miracle of Guru Ram Das had begun to unfold.

Notes

1. S. Premka Kaur; "Rejoinder", *Beads of Truth*, June 74

2. Dr. Shamsher Singh; *The Man Called the Siri Singh Sahib*, pg. 45

3. Yogi Bhajan; Khalsa Women's Training Camp 1983

4. Yogi Bhajan; *Beads of Truth*, Summer 1971

5. Yogi Bhajan

6. Gurcharn Singh Khalsa(Journalist); *The Man Called the Siri Singh Sahib*, pg. 40

7. Yogi Bhajan; Khalsa Women's Training Camp lecture, July 26, 1990

8. Yogi Bhajan; *Beads of Truth*, June 1973

9. Yogi Bhajan; *Man to Man,* 1978

10. Shakti Parwha Kaur; *Beads of Truth*, June 73

11. Yogi Bhajan; *Beads of Truth*, Summer 1971

12. Yogi Bhajan; *Beads of Truth*, December 1972

13. Yogi Bhajan; *Beads of Truth*, Winter Solstice 1973

14. Khalsa & Khalsa, editors; *The Man Called the Siri Singh Sahib*, pg. 71

15. *Shiromani Gurdwara Parbandhak Committee-* The chief management body for the Sikhs

16. Shakti Parwha Kaur Khalsa; *The Man Called the Siri Singh Sahib*, pg. 117

17. Yogi Bhajan; *Beads of Truth*, Fall 1980

18. Yogi Bhajan: Khalsa Women's Training Camp lecture 1982

19. Yogi Bhajan; *Beads of Truth*, December 1972

20. Yogi Bhajan; *Beads of Truth*, Fall 1975

21. Although purchased by Yogi Bhajan with money earned from teaching, he later donated the building to the ownership of Sikh Dharma.

22. *Beads of Truth*, March 1973

23. *Beads of Truth*, June 1973

24. Shakti Parwha Kaur; *Beads of Truth*, December 1972

25. Khalsa & Khalsa, Editors, *The Man Called the Siri Singh Sahib* pg. 108

26. Yogi Bhajan ; *Beads of Truth*, Fall 1977

Guru of Miracles
by S.S. Gurutej Singh Khalsa

The streets of Goindwal you walked alone,
Selling your pulses to stay alive,
A simple orphan, trying to survive,
Then Guru called you into His home.
And you, afraid and insecure,
Began to cry because you were unsure
If this experience you would survive.

But Guru in His mercy, took you in
And Bibi Bani he made your wife,
To inspire you through your trials of life,
But there was still more for you to win.
So he raised and tested and hammered you,
He found your heart pure then crowned you Guru,
Then you cut through Maya's veil like a knife.

Three sons were born, through darkness and light,
Though Prithi Chand's deception betrayed your trust,
And you were forced to dismiss him with disgust,
Still, there was Arjan, your heart's delight.
His longing for the Guru, sweet and pure,
Was fulfilled when you set your signature,
For the Guruship, to him, did you entrust.

You gave the world the Sarovar,
To wash away the wounds of the Soul,
Where we, who are broken, are restored whole,
And those who are defeated, start over.
Then in it, the Harimandir was placed,
Where all who bow are touched by Thy Grace
And those who have longings are consoled.

To guide us in marriage you wrote the Lavan,
To give us direction and see us through
Our lives should orbit around the Guru,
And in our souls, two hearts should beat as One.
For it is in the cozy home that God is found,
Where Grace and Dignity and Love abound,
Where life, itself, can be renewed.

Your beloved son came and bowed at your door
And prayed that you take his powers away,
That his ego should fly and his soul be saved,
Then, nightly for four years, he washed your floor.
But Guru's prophecy was to be fulfilled,
So you sent that son with the iron will
To carry your banner and show the way.

And here, in the West, a few were found
Who heard the Miracle of the Fourth Guru,
Who laid the foundation upon which we grew,
It is here that your praises resound.
Many lives have been touched by your hand
And by Thy Grace we continue to expand
And our hearts, you continue to imbue.

Oh, Guru of Miracles, before you we pray,
That we should remember, when lost and dark,
That our way is illumined by Guru's arc
And through you we will find the way.
For this is the Miracle of the Fourth Guru;
That you hold our course, straight and true,
And your son, the Yogi, has chiseled that spark.

Chapter Two

Establishing the Ministry of Sikh Dharma 1972-1974

*I*n the days of Guru Gobind Singh, the most talented and spiritually enlightened peo-ple sat in the Guru's court. One day, a simpleton named Bela came to Guru Gobind Singh and requested to be a student.

As the days went by, the simple and devoted Bela worked in the Guru's stable taking care of his horses and studied each day with the Guru. It so happened that Guru Gobind Singh and his soldiers had to leave to fight a lengthy military engagement, and so the Guru told Bela that he would not be able to teach him again until he returned. "Then we shall study tomorrow," said Bela. "Oh Bela," exclaimed the Guru lovingly, "Tera vakat na vela!" "You have no sense of time!"

During the months that the Guru was gone, Bela faithfully meditated on the Guru's last words "no sense of time," and by the grace of his one-pointed devotion, Bhai Bela experienced the ecstasy of God consciousness.

When Guru Gobind Singh returned, he saw the beautiful aura of spiritual enlight-enment that surrounded Bhai Bela, and so he invited him to sit in the Guru's presence. The other members of the court were jealous and complained to the Guru, "Why is it that a simpleton can achieve such spiritual distinction, and we who are so learned and have served for so long cannot?" The Guru replied, "You have been with me and served me well, but you have never really imbibed my words. Only those who meditate on the words of the Guru with singular devotion will know the mysteries of the unknown."

The Birth of a Nation

Nineteen seventy-two was an exciting time of growth, optimism, and high spirits for Sikh Dharma ashrams across the United States, Central and South American, Canada, Europe, and Japan. Firmly established, they were continuing to grow at a rapid pace. Through the devotion and love of many students, the Guru Ram Das Ashrams prospered and expanded in size and scope. In almost every major city in the United States, one could see the white clothes, white turbans, and long, flowing beards of the western Khalsa. These Sikhs took their place in the community, as leaders and as active participants in community service projects.

In keeping with the teachings of Guru Nanak, the Siri Singh Sahib emphasized the importance of living a householder's life. He often said, **"God is not found on the mountain tops, He lives in cozy homes."** Most ashram heads were married, bringing an environment of stability and family to ashram life. Children were born, and the first generation of western Sikhs began to grow. A vision of the future as seen by Guru Gobind Singh began to crystallize.

Chhiaanve karor khaalsaa sajega
Khaalsaa raaj karegaa

960 million pure ones shall adopt the path of purity
And the pure ones shall rule

Sau Saakhee

Although still in its infancy, the Siri Singh Sahib saw this newborn organization as the manifestation of the Guru's vision. Crossing all borders and barriers of culture, Sikh Dharma was more than an organization, it was a nation of people, the Khalsa Spiritual Nation.

The flag of the nation of Sikh Dharma was designed in the spring of 1972, based on ancient tradition and future prophesy. It was during the 1972 Summer Solstice Sadhana in Mendocino, California, that the gold and white flag of Sikh Dharma of the Western Hemisphere was first raised by the sangat. "This flag represents the symbol for the emerging spirituality in the world today. The white triangle in the upper portion of the background represents the 'shanti' principle; the symbol of purity, light, peace, tranquility, harmony, and saintliness. The lower triangle of yellow represents the 'shakti' principle and symbolizes power, courage, sacrifice, and action. The yellow triangle supports the white, as action comes first before one achieves purity, for there is 'no liberation without labor and no freedom which is free.' The bold, blue Adi Shakti symbol in the center represents the logos of primal energy, the source of creativity and all of creation."[1]

Service to the Community

In the tradition established by the Sikh Gurus, community service held a high priority with the sangat. In Tucson, the Maha Deva Ashram opened the first 3HO Free Kitchen, serving food to everyone who came. During the first week they opened their doors, over 500 people came to share a meal of mung beans and rice, salad, home-baked whole wheat bread, and fruit. At first, young people who were hitchhiking through Tucson on their way across the highways of America were the people who filled the langar hall. But soon the word spread, and mothers, children, businessmen in suits, and university students started frequenting the kitchen to enjoy the good food and spiritual atmosphere. Long-haired hippies sat side-by-side with business executives in the tradition of the Guru's langar. At meal time, cars lined the street, bicycles were stacked outside, and dogs waited eagerly for their masters to leave the free kitchen. Music and laughter were in the air, and this became an exciting place where people could come to share healthy vegetarian food and plenty of good "Sat Nam" vibrations.

Under the direction of Krishna Kaur, the Guru Ram Das Ashram on Broadway in Los Angeles initiated many service projects for the underprivileged people of the city. Located in the heart of inner Los Angeles, the Broadway ashram offered a ray of light and hope to many. The ashram was comprised of two storefronts joined by a common backyard. One building was used as a live-in ashram where regular yoga classes were offered. The other section served as a children's school, making quality child care available to the area's residents. The ashram offered a free kitchen every Tuesday and Saturday. Krishna Kaur instituted many other ambitious community aid projects, including the "Sat Nam Street Players." This group of musicians went out into the troubled streets of the black ghetto in East Los Angeles to bring inspiration and positive alternatives to the street activities.

Throughout the country, the newly established Guru Ram Das Ashrams opened their doors to feed the hungry, uplift the downhearted, and give shelter to those who needed it. Just to walk into an ashram, with the spicy aroma of Yogi Tea brewing and the sound of Khalsa music playing, was enough to lift the spirits and lighten the heart.

Learning from a Spiritual Teacher
The Siri Singh Sahib recognized the immense responsibility given to him by God and Guru to teach, to lead, and to share his wisdom with every person who came into his sphere. Without prejudice, he related not to the personality of his students, but to the soul within them. He often said, **"If you cannot see God in all, you cannot see God at all."**

Few Americans had the experience of learning from a spiritual teacher. In that classic tradition, the Siri Singh Sahib was at once hard and soft, logical and irrational, attractive and repelling. He said, "That is how I gain trust with your hearts. I come right out and blow your mind. You never like it; you always avoid me. You do everything but I don't care. Whatever the situation is, I come right out and put a big cannon ball into you. This is what you have to learn to do: zero and let yourself go—your total self, not just a part of you!"

Sometimes he would yell with the force of a typhoon! Sometimes he would gently speak with the voice of a poet. Yet always he would bring the student around to the realization and awareness of the God within. He described his technique as **"Poke, provoke, confront, and elevate,"** taking a student beyond the limitations of the ego.

Once in Los Angeles, there was a sword on the altar that had a small piece of metal broken on the handle. In the manner of a spiritual teacher, he used this as a teaching tool to bring an inner awareness to his students. He chastised them, saying, "I want to know if you have seen the torn part of it. This sword has been torn. Do you see the unawareness of it? The darkness of the consciousness this represents? It represents that with two eyes we are blind. It represents that with all of our affection and devotion we are careless. It is my very humble prayer to you all to remember that your symbols, your homes, those things with which you've shared the joy of God consciousness should not be allowed to stay torn like this. Every action represents everything from and unto God. That is total consciousness, that is total awareness. It is an Infinity." [2]

As described by one of his early students: "What he knows only he knows. Who can know the depth of the man? From a distance he is imposing—his height, his white clothes and turban, a simple graceful man. Some feel distant from him. Some don't understand him. Some think they do. Some think they are his favorites and are close to him. But all are wrong, for he is universal in the true sense. He has no favorites, he has no enemies, he has no friends, he has no one but God. Students wait for his favors, he blesses them all and hassles anyone who can take it. Some feel lucky, some are disappointed, all are wrong. He loves everyone, but plays the game of life better than any. He is the same to all, for he sees nothing but God." [3]

The telephone became one of his most effective teaching tools—"213-273-9422" was an open line for students to call and speak directly to the Siri Singh Sahib, day or night. Doubts, fears, problems, and anxieties were all poured out over the phone line, and wisdom and spiritual reassurance from the Siri Singh Sahib were given back in large doses. Regardless of how busy he was, he still took the time to speak personally to everyone who called. After a busy day of teaching, administrating, and counseling, the Siri Singh Sahib would make phone calls into the early hours of the morning. It was not unusual to receive a call from him at 2:00 or 3:00 AM.

The Traveling Teacher

During the summer months of 1972, the teaching and travel schedule of the Siri Singh Sahib continued to escalate. With 3HO Ashrams all over the world, the leadership responsibilities of the Siri Singh Sahib and his staff became enormous. In June, July, and August of 1972, the Siri Singh Sahib toured Europe, visiting the 3HO Ashrams that he had established there. In London he had a full schedule of speaking engagements, press conferences, and an eight-day White Tantric Yoga Course held at the Guru Ram

Das Ashram in London. The Indian Sikhs in London were very curious about the presence of the western Sikhs, and were moved and inspired by the lectures of the Siri Singh Sahib. Being separated from India for more than a generation, they had found that they were losing their culture and were being absorbed into the western style of life. These sons and daughters of India found great inspiration in the youthful and vibrant student-teachers of the Siri Singh Sahib who were living the lifestyle of the Guru's teachings. This was the first of many "missionary" tours undertaken by Sikh Dharma.

A good friend of the Siri Singh Sahib's from his early years in India, Gurcharn Singh Khalsa had settled and established himself in England. A very well known journalist and respected Gursikh, Gurcharn Singh gave his full support to the mission of the western Khalsa. He later became a minister of Sikh Dharma of the Western Hemisphere, participated in the Khalsa Council, and served the sangat through his valued advice and talented writings.

From London, the Siri Singh Sahib traveled to Paris and continued with his teaching tour. Upon invitation from Pope Paul VI, the Siri Singh Sahib traveled to Rome for a private audience at the papal summer residence. In this meeting, Pope Paul and the Siri Singh Sahib discussed the possibility of convening a world spiritual conference in Rome under the guidance of the Pope. This idea did finally come to fruition under Pope John Paul II when the Vatican sponsored a huge prayer gathering in Assis, Italy in October 1986.

The Siri Singh Sahib returned from his first European tour in August, then departed again in September for a missionary tour of the Orient. He visited Tokyo and introduced Sikh Dharma to Japan in a series of classes and lectures. He spoke in the Hong Kong gurdwaras, urging the local sangat to return to the values and teachings of the Gurus. He finished his tour in Singapore, teaching every day at 5:00 AM at the Guru Nanak Sat Sang Sabha Gurdwara.

The Siri Singh Sahib continued to tour different segments of the United States, serving the needs of the western sangat and teaching White Tantric Yoga. In December of 1972, during his visit to the east coast, Shakti Parwha wrote the following about his itinerary: "On the east coast in early December, Yogi Bhajan lectured at Harvard University, MIT [Massachusetts Institute of Technology], The Unitarian Church of Hartford, University of Massachusetts, Smith College, and Amherst College, in addition to smaller group sessions with students and faculty, and of course our own centers in the various cities. There's no room to list even the itinerary, much less to fill in details of all the TV, radio, and press interviews. It's not easy, for the pace has accelerated, and the scope of Yogiji's mission is ever expanding, commensurate with the necessity of the times."[4]

It seemed that the Siri Singh Sahib was constantly traveling during this formative period of Sikh Dharma, leading his people by walking in the front. In 1973, he spent more than 170 days "on the road"; teaching, inspecting, administrating, and inspiring.

"Once upon a time, the spiritual teacher, the holy man, trudged on foot to spread his message of Truth. Or else, he sat upon a deerskin in the forest beside his hut, and the faithful and the curious came to listen and stayed to pray. But in this machine age, answering the urgency of the times, by car, by plane, by helicopter, Yogi Bhajan reaches and preaches!"[5]

The Form and Structure of Sikh Dharma in the West

The Siri Singh Sahib understood that for Sikh Dharma of the Western Hemisphere to survive the tests and challenges that lay ahead, a clear and strong organizational structure was required. Sikh Dharma needed a form that would serve the coming generations, beyond the realm of personality and politics. In recognition of this, in January, 1972 the Siri Singh Sahib ordained the first men and women to serve as ministers of Sikh Dharma in a ceremony in Los Angeles. He gave them the distinguished titles of "Singh Sahib" and "Sardarni Sahiba," charging them with the responsibility for the welfare of the sangat in their respective areas. Increasingly, more and more people were attracted to Sikh Dharma, bringing with them the pain and confusion endemic to western society. Ministers were needed to counsel and support people, serving the sangat in every big and small way. A minister in Sikh Dharma was not a post of status or power, but one of humility and service. A minister did not hold a status higher than that of any other Gursikh; rather, he or she was considered a servant of the sangat.

Because Sikh Dharma was spread over a vast geographic area, the Sikh Dharma centers were grouped into regions with the largest ashram in the area designated as the Regional Center. Each Regional Center was administered by a Regional Director and a Regional Secretary. The Regional Centers assumed full responsibility for the welfare of the people within their area.

The Regional Centers were served and administrated by Sikh Dharma International Headquarters in Los Angeles. The letters and phone calls continued to pour into Los Angeles as Sikh Dharma rapidly grew. "In three and one-half years our 3HO family has grown from an idea in the mind of God and expressed to us by Yogi Bhajan, to more than 108 ashrams and over 150,000 students!"[6] As a result of this growth, the Siri Singh Sahib expanded his office staff to better meet the needs of the sangat. In 1972, Shakti Parwha Kaur served as Executive Secretary; Sardarni Premka Kaur, Administrative Director; Sat Simran Kaur, Director of Public Relations; Gurumeet Kaur, Office Secretary; and Nirinjan Kaur, Personal Secretary.

The Siri Singh Sahib established the positions of "Mukhia Singh Sahib" and "Mukhia Sardarni Sahiba" to create a leadership body for the Sikh Dharma ministry. These ministers were drawn from the Regional Directors and the prominent administrative leaders of Sikh Dharma International. The Siri Singh Sahib established them as the "Council of the Khalsa," the beginnings of what was later to become the Khalsa Council, and together they sat to discuss and develop their roles as leaders in this emerging Khalsa Nation.

In order to fully establish Sikh Dharma in the West, the Siri Singh Sahib successfully worked to have Sikhism recognized as a religion by the United States Government. The corporate By-laws and Articles of Incorporation for Sikh Dharma were draft-ed, establishing the organization as a legal religious entity. These documents were endorsed on April 10, 1973 by the State of California. On May 17, 1973, the Federal Government recognized Sikh Dharma as a religion, granting them the privileges and protection enjoyed by other churches across America.

On October 23, 1974, the Siri Singh Sahib drafted the "Principles of the Dharma" in which he outlined the qualifications and definition of a Sikh in clear, straightforward English. This document has served the many ashrams and teachers spreading the teachings of Guru Nanak, giving them a distinct and consolidated standard from which to instruct the many people who came to their classes.

Khalsa Family Businesses

Many Sikhs started their own businesses to employ and support themselves and the young people living in the ashrams. The first "family business" was the Sunshine Brass Bed Factory in Los Angeles. Under the leadership of Guru Singh, this business pros-pered and helped establish the Los Angeles Sikh Dharma community. For the people who worked in the family businesses, it was more than just a job, they were working toward a common goal of strength and stability for Sikh Dharma.

"By ones and twos we arrive at the Brass Bed Factory, all seven of us ready to begin another day. But the event of our coming together is not just a few men going to work in Los Angeles. There is something very special about it, a special warmth and a special purpose. Shortly, we are all standing together in a circle—holding hands in the middle of the brass and the benches and singing and chanting together, a practice we do each day. As we chant, I am reminded that what we are doing is something bigger than just building a business, something bigger than just making money, some-thing bigger than any material thing. I am aware that we are living out an ideal, find-ing a way to live in peace and harmony."[7]

One of the most enterprising early business ventures was the Golden Temple Conscious Cookery Restaurants. The unique feature of the restaurants was not only the delightful and plentiful vegetarian food, but the attitude of the people who were serving there. For them, work was a sadhana, a spiritual offering of service, and therefore they met the public with an attitude of love and the vibration of "Sat Nam." Many people patronized the Golden Temple Restaurants as much to feed their souls as to feed their stomachs. By early 1973, there were 12 Golden Temple Conscious Cookery Restaurants throughout the world, in Washington, DC, Amsterdam, London, Los Angeles, Tucson, Phoenix, Boston, Ottawa, Toronto, Kansas City, Denver, and Santa Fe.

The first Golden Temple Conscious Cookery was opened in Washington, DC in the spring of 1972. The restaurant provided a strong foundation for the students in the ashram and they no longer had to find work outside the 3HO community. Youthful exuberance combined with a total lack of business experience made for long working hours and great sacrifices on the part of the restaurant workers. Nonetheless, the restaurants were very popular and prospered for the benefit of all.

"Under the pressures of shorthandedness and inexperience, the restaurant was the teacher that brought the members of Ahimsa Ashram into their first practical experience of group consciousness. The extended daily schedule pushed the restaurant workers to the point where they felt they could work no more—the point where they were *sure* they could work no more, and then to the point where they had forgotten themselves and were indeed working longer and harder. Each night at closing time, the tired but cheerful crew assembled in front of the restaurant and locked arms, bound with that love that is a blessing to those who have worked together for something they believe in. They would sway, laugh, dance, and sing out a song of ecstasy: *Ek Ong Kar Sat Nam Siri Wha Guru!* Then with the mind and body cleared of the day's tensions and efforts, they would return to the kitchen again for another three or four hours of clean-up."[8]

After going home to sleep and meditate, they would go back the next day to the restaurant to do it all again. Amazingly enough, all the Golden Temple Restaurants throughout the world shared the same type of scenario for the sevadars who served in them.

The Guru Ram Das Ashram in Eugene, Oregon was a pioneer in the health food industry of the Pacific Northwest. Baking in a small commercial kitchen, the people of the ashram sold delicious whole wheat bread, apple cakes, and granola from what was then called the Amrit Bakery. Always a lover of sweets, one of the Sikhs came up with a recipe for a chewy candy made from honey and nuts left over from a day of baking. In a quote from Guru Ram Das, it is written, "With every breath, and with every bite of food, remember to utter *Wha Guru*," so in honor of Guru Ram Das, the bakers named the candy bar "Wha Guru Chew." This tasty candy was a big success since it was made from healthy and wholesome ingredients. At first, the Wha Guru Chew was sold locally along with the bakery products, but soon it was picked up by a national distributor and began appearing in health food stores across the county. This was the first 3HO product to be distributed nationally, and is still a favorite today. "Son," the Siri Singh Sahib said many years later, "When you and I are long gone, the Wha Guru Chew will still be here!"

At the direction of the Siri Singh Sahib, Mutka Kaur instituted a drug rehabilitation program based on the 3HO teachings at the Maha Deva Ashram in Tucson, Arizona. By taking young people who were addicted to heroin and other narcotics into the ashram and away from the street, the program was able to give them a cleansing and healthy diet, restore their health through Kundalini Yoga, and teach them the self-control of meditation. The 3HO Drug Rehabilitation Program realized incredible success and was soon in the top 10 percent of effective drug rehabilitation programs in America. They went on to be federally funded and accredited by the United States Government.

A Letter From a Client of the 3HO Drug Rehabilitation Program

*T*he logical beginning of any great event is birth. In my case, let's call it a re-birth. No one could have been more displaced and negative during my first days at the Maha Deva Ashram. But, as the lesser of two evils, my wife and I packed it in and swallowed the pill. As I sit here on upon my mat contemplating certain events over the past few weeks, it is most difficult to find the proper expression - the problem being that there does not exist within my vocabulary adequate words to express my state of mind (I should say, state of spirit). Only God knows the essence of dependency of a heroin addict, but as I begin to experience the God in me, it is only logical that dependency should fall away.

I will stay here until my growing is finished. My heart is light, my smile is sure, and my confidence is growing. One week ago today, an old friend quickly slammed closed the trunk of his car after I undauntedly refused a sampling of his "portable drugstore." He stared fixedly into my eyes and shook my hand. Ole Joe ain't what he used to be. Thank God!

March 12, 1973

The First Gurdwara in the Guru Ram Das Ashram

When the Guru Ram Das Ashram in Los Angeles was first established, there were Sunday morning services called "Scriptures of the World." Here, inspirational readings and lectures were presented by different speakers and the group joined together in singing their own compositions of spiritual songs. But as the young Sikhs gained more experience from the Guru's teachings, they learned to read from the *Siri Guru Granth Sahib* and play Gurbani Kirtan. From the love and devotion radiating from their hearts, their Sunday program transformed into traditional Sikh Gurdwara services. The first Gurdwara at the Guru Ram Das Ashram in Los Angeles was held when the Siri Singh Sahib was out of town. The men from the Brass Bed Factory built a beautiful Palki Sahib in brass and installed the *Siri Guru Granth Sahib* in the main sadhana room. November 26, 1972, marked the date of the first Sunday Gurdwara service held in Guru Ram Das Ashram on Preuss Road.

The Siri Singh Sahib was away from Los Angeles on a teaching tour for the first few Sundays and this gave the students about a month to work out all the details. American Sikh songs were played on the guitar and some simple Gurbani Kirtan shabads were played on the harmonium. Ardas was read from the *Peace Lagoon,* and the hukam was read in both Gurmukhi and English.

When the Siri Singh Sahib attended the first Gurdwara at the ashram, he was amazed and humbled by the miracle that had been created in his absence.

"There are very few people who have had the experience of imagining a thing and then one morning getting up and seeing that thing actually happening. This is not the privilege of all people. But sometimes it happens that a man like me, who never understood who God is, who perhaps only had a belief that there is a Guru, and that the love of Guru may have been so strong that God might have wanted to show me He exists. So, He has, in His Grace, created a creativity that is most astonishing for me to behold!"[9]

Soon all the larger ashrams held Gurdwara services on Sunday morning, bringing together the western Sikhs as well as the Indian born Sikhs in love and service to the *Siri Guru Granth Sahib.*

His Family Arrives From India

After going through the long, drawn out formalities of obtaining permanent resident status, the Siri Singh Sahib was able to arrange for his wife and family to come to the United States. The three years they had waited in India had been a long and difficult sacrifice. When they packed up their belongings to come to the United States, it was with trepidation for they had no idea what to expect. Finally in 1972, Bibiji Inderjit Kaur joined Yogi Bhajan in America with their three children.

Although Bibiji had met several of the western Sikhs in India, she found the situation in America surprising. The sangat was very young and she met many students who were still hippies, just starting out on the path of self-awareness. Bibiji traveled extensively with the Siri Singh Sahib, teaching the basics of Sikh Dharma in the ashrams across the United States. She instructed people in the proper pronunciation and translations of the Sikh daily banis and in the care and protocol of the *Siri Guru Granth Sahib.* She was a role model for the many Sikh women who were new wives and mothers in Sikh Dharma.

In September, 1973 the Siri Singh Sahib's father, Dr. Kartar Singh Puri, came from India to visit his son in America. "Papaji," as he was affectionately called by the students of 3HO, stayed for a while in the ashram in Española to teach Punjabi and Sikh history. He soon became a well known figure in the town of Española as he walked five miles each day to maintain his health. He would wave to all the neighbors, and take a few moments to stop and chat, coming in for a cup of tea. For many years after Papaji returned to India, local people would ask about him.

Throughout his life Papaji maintained his personal sadhana of reciting the Sukhmani Sahib twice a day. When the Siri Singh Sahib was seven years old, he became very ill with measles, complicated with dysentery and a severe ear infection. Papaji brought him to Amritsar to see a doctor but as the illness progressed, the hope of recovery began to fade. Sitting in meditation, Papaji prayed for the mercy of Guru Ram Das to spare the life of young Harbhajan. If only he would recover, Papaji pledged to recite Sukhmani daily in thanksgiving for the kindness and greatness of God. When Papaji returned to his son's bedside, Harbhajan looked up into the worried face of his father and said, "Guru Ram Das has appeared to me and he has told me what can cure my sickness. If your medicine has all been tried, then you should now give me the medicine which I suggest. Let me drink the juice of two onions and let an onion be fried in oil and that oil, when it is just warm, should be dropped into my ear." Papaji immediately did as his son said, and through the mercy of Guru Ram Das the illness began to disappear. In gratitude and thanksgiving, from that day onward Papaji recited not one but two Sukhmani Sahibs daily.

For the benefit of the young Sikhs, Papaji translated the Sukhmani Sahib into English, and many sat with him during his recitation. He patiently explained the meaning of each stanza, igniting the love of Guru in their hearts.

Returning to India in February, 1973

The Siri Singh Sahib's eldest son, Ranbir Singh, went to school in Phoenix, Arizona and lived there in the ashram. In February, 1973, his two younger children, Kamaljit Kaur and Kulbir Singh, returned to school in India at the Guru Nanak Fifth Centenary School in Mussoorie. Sarab Shakti Kaur and Darian Drew joined them, and were the first Sikh children from the West to obtain their education there. Under the Sikh Dharma Foreign Education program, hundreds of western children have since attended school in India.

Bibiji set off to India with her two children in February 1973, taking with her a small group of 3HO ladies and Dale Singh Sklar (who became the first Bhai Sahib of Sikh Dharma, Bhai Sahib Dayal Singh). During that first month the group spent in New Delhi, the ladies learned to play a few shabads on the harmonium. Soon word spread about the "Amrikan Bibis," and Ganga Bhajan Kaur, Sat Kirn Kaur, Dr. Sat Kirpal Kaur, and Ram Das Kaur played simple but devotional Gurbani Kirtan in gurdwaras all over Delhi. They were the object of a great deal of respect as well as curiosity, for as the Siri Singh Sahib had promised, the American Sikhs were returning to India to inspire the Indians themselves. In this way the sangat was reminded of the true meaning of the teachings of the Sikh Gurus; many were inspired to live the Rehit again, growing their hair and beards and tying their turbans. Bahadur Singh was the Siri Singh Sahib's 3HO representative in India, and he worked tirelessly to serve the jatha and make arrangements for kirtan programs.

On April 9, 1973, the group joined the Guru Gobind Singh Mahan Yatra, celebrating the inauguration of the newly built Guru Gobind Singh Marg, a highway linking 91 historical sites and 222 villages associated with the life of Guru Gobind Singh. Giani Zail Singh, who was then the Chief Minister of Punjab, guided and cared for the group. Under his direction, they visited and played kirtan at all the gurdwaras along the 640-kilometer route. They were received with an enthusiastic response from the sangat and thousands of people joined in the singing. Giani Zail Singh later went on to be the President of India, maintaining a close relationship with the western Sikhs, guiding and counseling them with his unique perspective and wisdom.

Though their mission in India was momentous, it is important to remember that this group was mostly comprised of bright, energetic young people in their late teens and early twenties. In a letter to the Siri Singh Sahib from Gurucharan Kaur, this youthful exuberance is delightfully illustrated:

In India, Hola Mahela is a festive religious holiday celebrated in the spring. Known as the "day of colors," young people roam the streets aggressively throwing small bags of colored water on each other, creating a big mess and a lot of fun. At Dam Dama Sahib, the gurdwara where the jatha was staying, Hola Mahela was quite a holiday.

"Outside the refuge of the gurdwara, colors, dyes, paints, and water were being thrown all over everyone. We tried to avoid getting caught in the play but when Charan Pal arrived here with colors and having five young energetic teenagers in our home, we bowed to the inevitable. It is quite a sight to see graceful American ladies smeared with multicolored dyes and soaking wet. Even those of us who barricaded themselves in the living room were not spared.

"Just as we were about to leave for a second round of play, we received a call from Bahadur Singh saying we had to be at the Gurdwara Dam Dama Sahib in 30 minutes to present kirtan! This was quite a surprise. There was a great flurry of scrubbing, changing, combing, and a group which 30 minutes earlier had looked a mess, emerged shining white and ready to represent 3HO Grace of God.

"With a few thousand people staring at us, we presented the two shabads that we have learned and practiced. Even though our rhythm was a little off, the sangat was surprised, pleased, excited, and warmly receptive. We were each presented with a garland of flowers while cries of "Bole So Nihal" were heard from all directions.

"Dale Singh [who was 19 years old at the time], stood and made a small speech that said briefly: 'Don't be surprised to see American Sikhs. Within many of your lifetimes you will see Sikhs from all countries. It is our prayer that they will live in the brotherhood of the Khalsa as Guru Gobind Singh has instructed. The *Siri Guru Granth Sahib* will be translated into every language in the world.' This was met with much approval."[10]

When the jatha traveled to Amritsar, the Sarvoar (the tank of water surrounding the Golden Temple) was drained and Kar Seva was in process. The travelers from America participated in cleaning out the mud and silt that had collected on the bottom of the tank. This is a great event that is done every 50 years, so only once in a person's lifetime does this blessed opportunity come. Together with the Sikhs of Amritsar, the American jatha collected the mud and carried it out in baskets on their heads. Their white clothes became dark and soiled, but their souls became luminous with the love of Guru Ram Das. As Gurucharan Kaur writes: "Each time I go to the Golden Temple and listen to the kirtan, or maybe just bow to Guruji, I cry. It is a feeling that is very difficult to describe. I don't want anything ... just that His presence form a warm blanket over me. This emotion merges into devotion, and I wish to serve in any way possible. I have never felt stronger, more fearless, more loving, more beautiful ever before in my life. I want to embrace the whole world and give them water from my fingertips." Moved by the love of Guru Ram Das, many of the group received the blessing of Amrit from the Akal Takhat.

After leaving the school children in Mussoorie, the jatha returned to America in May, bringing with them the new gift of being able to play Gurbani Kirtan, and the intense devotion and love for Guru Ram Das. These two blessings served to shape and guide the western Sikhs from that time onward.

Bhai Sahib Dayal Singh

Some of the young people who were drawn to the ashram seemed to have an innate affinity for the historical writings, script, and language of the Sikhs. In an amazingly short period of time, they assimilated and mastered the technology and philosophy of the Sikh Gurus. One such person was Dayal Singh, who came to the Guru Ram Das Ashram in Los Angeles at the age of 16. He was a young man with an extraordinary capacity for seva, and a exceptional love for Guru. During his visit to India in February, he was permeated with a profound attitude of devotion that he carried back to the sangat in the United States. He learned to write and understand Gurmukhi script, so he was the first western Khalsa to be able to read and translate the *Siri Guru Granth Sahib* for others. In June, 1973, in recognition of the advanced soul of this young man, the Siri Singh Sahib ordained Dayal Singh as the Head Granthi for the Sikh Dharma of the Western Hemisphere. At the age of 19 years, Dayal Singh was given the title of "Bhai Sahib." Bhai Sahib Dayal Singh worked tirelessly in spreading the teachings of the Gurus throughout the young sangat in America. "Bhai Sahib shared all he knew with all those who came to learn, giving classes in Gurmukhi, translating Gurbani and instructing everyone in the proper care of the *Siri Guru Granth Sahib*. Many began to know and love Bhai Sahib in a way they had never done before."[11]

Baisakhi Day is always an important event, but April 13, 1974 in Los Angeles was a remarkable day. Sant Mihan Singh had come from India with several of his Sikhs to visit and serve the western sangat. In the pre-dawn hours at Guru Ram Das Ashram in Los Angeles, they administered Amrit to dozens of American Sikhs. Bhai Sahib Dayal Singh was one of the Punj Piare, and this was the first time a western Sikh had served in this role. Standing in the dim light, this young man took his place with the gray-bearded and very respected Gursikhs from India.

Summer Solstice Sadhana

Summer Solstice Sadhana was an exciting time of year. From all over the world people came by car, by plane, and by bus for the annual reunion of 3HO. Separated by oceans and continents, this was the only time of year many friends had the chance to see each other. People worked and saved their money all year to be able to attend Summer and Winter Solstices. It was a time of renewal, growth, and inspiration.

In the summer of 1973, Summer Solstice Sadhana was held in New Mexico, in the Jemez Mountains. Over 1,000 people attended the camp and the spiritual energy of the sangat was electric. "Guru Gobind Singh's prophecy of a new Khalsa showed its character as the 3HO family, for its fourth consecutive year, celebrated our annual Summer Solstice Sadhana amidst the splendors of a New Mexico mountain setting. The 7,500-foot altitude furnished the tests over which we strove to triumph: water shortages, frosty nights, sultry days, torrential downpours, and oxygen-thin air. Nevertheless, as a family, our spirit and unity proved themselves to courageously overcome physical hardships and we joyously praised the One Creator amidst it all."[12]

Each day began at 4:00 AM with morning sadhana, Ardas, and flag-raising. On the second day, the rule of "silence" descended on the camp, and only the sound of "Wahe Guru" was to be heard. During the eight days of silence, White Tantric Yoga began at 11:00 AM, and continued to 5:00 or 6:00 PM, depending on the results of the group as determined by the Mahan Tantric. In the evenings, the talented musicians of Sikh Dharma came together to sing and the entire camp participated with joyous hearts. On the tenth day the vow of silence lifted, and the camp came alive with Gurdwara, Sikh vows, and marriages. In 1973, over 200 ministers were ordained, and took vows to selflessly serve the sadh sangat.

"These ten days are filled with labor; the labor of love, of serving our entire family in a more direct way. Sometimes that labor may mean working in the kitchen, cleaning the huge pots, and chopping mountains of vegetables. Sometimes it may include a day in Children's Camp, with nearly 200 new 3HO babies and children to take care of. A day's work might also include serving food at meal time, carrying large containers of oranges, bananas, and hot soup up and down the row upon row of healthy, happy, and holy people who have just completed an exhilarating and inspiring morning sadhana. But work doesn't just mean physical labor; it also means working on the Self, and that is really what Summer Solstice time means to the students and student-teachers who come to share these ten days in silence, in a disciplined lifestyle."[13]

The Khalsa String Band

After the energetic and inspiring music at Summer Solstice, the Sikh musicians of the "Khalsa String Band" decided to record an album. Although several of the members had done home recorded tapes, this time they would record their songs in a real music studio in New York City. Guruka Singh, who worked at National Studios, set up the session and they gathered in New York City to cut the album "Spiritual Nation."

"We came from all over this county. Some drove at 90 miles per hour to get there, other of us flew at six times that speed. We came broke, we came full, we came packing everything and nothing, we came with a lot of love and a lot of songs (many more than we could have possibly recorded) and charged with so much energy that we practically blew the lid off our serene ashram in Brooklyn where we all stayed. But you know that Kundalini and shakti energy, when it is channeled into God and Divine Consciousness—Wha Guru! It'll blow your head off too! So now we are a bunch of headless musicians, bowed and humble. We stand before God knowing that it is by His Grace, and His Grace alone, that we are used as instruments of His music."[14] The "Spiritual Nation" was a big success, selling out of the first release. The Khalsa String Band went on tour with the Siri Singh Sahib, and many of the radio stations across America started playing "Sat Nam" music.

3HO Continues to Unfold

In June of 1973, the Siri Singh Sahib bought a residence at 1905 Preuss Road in Los Angeles and the work of refurbishing it into the Guru Ram Das Estate was begun. By September of 1973, the work was completed, and Sikh Dharma had a place of grace and elegance in which to entertain guests and dignitaries. Congressmen, Senators, Ambassadors, Yogis, and Swamis were each received and shown the grace and hospitality of the House of Guru Ram Das.

3HO on the east coast continued to expand and grow with Washington, DC as the Regional Headquarters. Gurujot Kaur, who was the Regional Secretary writes: "The Siri Singh Sahib has been stressing that now is the time for expansion and growth. We must reach out to our communities and spread our beautiful message of 'Sat Nam' far and wide. We cannot relax and wait for people to come to us, but we must be the initiators. 'No time for hanging around in the bliss.' Yogiji has told us many times that we are the pioneers of the New Age and that it is our job to change the direction of the times. To what more Divine purpose can a man devote his life than to serve the humanity and to build a new nation based on selflessness and sacrifice, love and devotion."[15]

The Ahimsa Ashram had spread out among five residences with the house on Q Street as the spiritual center and the restaurant office complex as the organizational center. As Ahimsa grew, several measures were adopted to maintain the continuity of a spiritual ashram. Under the direction of Gurujot Singh, they formed the first Ashram Council. This committee of 12 members represented the diverse aspects of ashram life, serving to guide the management of the ashram.

In Pomona, Gurucharan Singh had developed a research center for a more scientific approach to Kundalini Yoga. The Kundalini Research Institute (KRI) performed a variety of experiments, documenting the effects of Kundalini Yoga and the 3HO lifestyle. In conducting research with healing kriyas, he experimented with the effects that meditation can have in the healing process. "From a group of unhealthy onion seedlings, Gurucharan Singh took one group and used healing kriyas on them while Gurubanda Singh watched a control group. Conditions for both groups were exactly the same except for the kriyas. The experiment was carried on for five days, 20 minutes a day. The results were amazing! The cells on the 'kriya seedlings' had reproduced more than twice as much as the control group!"[16]

KRI served as the collection point for the hundreds of lectures, yoga classes, and meditations taught by the Siri Singh Sahib each year. The staff of KRI transcribed the miles of tape generated by the Siri Singh Sahib and published these lectures in book form. The extensive documentation and publication of Kundalini Yoga classes by KRI allowed student-teachers to disseminate this vital information in their own classes. In 1974 they published "Sadhana Guidelines" in the *KRI Journal of Science and Consciousness*. Republished as a book in 1976, it is still a best-seller today.

The practice of sadhana was always the focal point of ashram life. During the first year or so, sadhana consisted of two and one-half hours of chanting "Ek Ong Kar Sat Nam Siri Wahe Guru" in the proper technology and method. Sadhana slowing evolved under the Siri Singh Sahib's direction to include other prayers and mantras, and it became a tradition to announce the new sadhana format at Summer Solstice.

Sadhana in the early 1970s

For the five or six people in our small ashram in New England, sadhana was the central and most important part of our day. We took turns being the wake-up person, which means that you woke up by the alarm clock at 3:00 AM. You would then gently wake the other people in the ashram by singing or chanting and knocking on their door. An icy cold shower at that hour of the morning was a real act of faith, but if you were serious about not falling asleep during the meditation, it was an essential part of the morning routine. Dressed in loose cotton clothes, we would all be in the sadhana room by 3:45 AM to read Japji together. In those days, none of us could read Gurmukhi, so we read the beautiful words of Japji in English from the Peace Lagoon, *like a lover whispering to her beloved. One of us would lead the group in a very energetic yoga set. The more difficult the exercises were, the better it was, trying to out-do each other in perfection of each posture and breath. Then sitting on our sheepskins with straight spines, wrapped in a favorite blanket, we began chanting "Long Ek Ong Kar's:"* Ek Ong Kar Sat Nam Siri Wahe Guru. *This morning chant was 62 minutes long, and if you didn't apply a serious effort of concentration you would fall asleep. But when you did it with the proper technique and concentration, you became charged with an electric energy and the vastness of the entire universe would be exposed to your head and heart. Sadhana did not seem long; it had a unique quality of absolute timelessness. When the meditation was finished we would inhale deeply, and then relax, lying down with our blankets covering us. Our consciousness was free to float high above our physical body. Sometimes we'd lose track of time and sleep for an hour or more! But normally we rested for about 15 minutes. Then we would chant to Guru Ram Das with a pure love and* *devotion. Before ending sadhana, the leader would read a hukam from the* Peace Lagoon, *and we would sing "May the Long Time Sun Shine Upon You." One of the ladies would bring in Yogi Tea and blanched almonds from the kitchen, and we smiled, relaxed, and enjoyed the company of each other briefly before dashing off to work somewhere. It was like nothing else I had ever experienced, and I waited all day to do it again the next morning.*

The Rehit of Guru Gobind Singh

When Guru Gobind Singh, the tenth Sikh Guru, established the order of the Khalsa in 1699, he established a clear discipline and code of conduct, a "Rehit," for his Sikhs to follow. This Rehit was based on practical and scientific teachings, and the western Sikhs adopted this discipline wholeheartedly in their dress and personal habits.

"The experiment of standing out was started and carried out by Guru Gobind Singh. He said that whosoever shall relate to the very spirit, and whose mind shall relate to the spirit, that body must represent it also. The body must represent it and be totally disciplined. Other than the discipline, he said, there is no relationship with me. And then openly he said:

> *Rehit piaaree mujh ko,*
> *Sikh piaaraa naahe*
>
> *Dear to me is the discipline of the Sikh,*
> *not the one who calls himself a Sikh."*[17]
>
> Rehit Nama by Bhai Desa Singh

The Khalsa of Guru Gobind Singh wore long, uncut hair, the *keshas.* The Siri Singh Sahib explained to his students that the hair on the human body serves a vital role in maintaining one's energy balance. Like an antenna, a person's hair acts as a conduit of energy impulses and will strengthen and constantly rejuvenate the electromagnetic field.

"If a person, from birth to the end, does not ruin the antenna of his hair, then insanity cannot come near that person. Guru Gobind Singh told you to keep it intact because there is a reason to God's scheme. There is a role this hair sitting on your head has to play. He knew that without this hair, you will go weak later in life.

"Guru Gobind Singh also told you to keep a *kanga*, a wooden comb. He was the most scientific of all scientists. He gave you the wooden comb so that you would create your own electric energy for your brain by combing your hair. When the sun is up, tie this kundal, a hair knot on top of your head, which Samson talks about in the Bible. Like Samson of the Old Testament, maintaining your hair is critical to your strength of body and mind.

"Then, to protect these antenna and your higher centers from the direct solar energy, you must cover your head with a turban. More than just a loose cotton cloth, a perfectly wrapped turban will set the moving plates of the skull, adjusting them into perfect alignment as required by a person of God. The word *Khalsa* has no gender. Male and female have exactly the same standard with respect to divinity and God's nature. In Khalsa there is no woman and there is no man. It is the purity of God. It is the form and shape of Guru Gobind Singh as he saw in his divinity. There are not separate rules for each. Hair, comb, and turban are requirements for all people, not just for men.

"He made you to wear *kachera*, underwear that creates its own air pocket over the thigh and the first four vertebrae of the spine. It is designed so that when you walk, it presses the legs in an area called the calcium area. That tiny underwear you wear is just like a fig leaf! He took you out of the fig leaf and made you to wear kachera so that the polarity of the second chakra, in the movement of the second chakra correlative to the nostrils, ida and pingala,[18] can be maintained by itself. In this way a person can enjoy his creative energy in life.

"He gave you the *kara*, a steel or iron bangle, to wear. On your right hand he gave you this sign, a sign to each other of slavery and freedom. He made you a slave to God so that you could be free of every other restriction. And the kara is a good tool as well. In battle, the kara will protect the fragile and flexible points of the wrist.

"Sometimes you ask me, 'Why do we wear a sword?' Guru Gobind Singh was the most wise human. He was the one wise human on this planet who knew not only the psychology of man, but the instincts of man. If you are asked to worship the arm, then you will respect it. You will never misuse it. He made it binding on your to wear a *kirpan*, a small sword, because it is the symbol of all weapons. When you worship the sword, you will be the last one to use a weapon. You will be the most sober and restrictive. You cannot play madly with something you worship. Have you ever seen any man, in his madness, throw his altar out of the window? Never. Guru Gobind Singh made us soldier-saints. This was a new formula, a blend of the saint and the soldier, a helper who never gives up."[19]

Sikh Dharma and the United States Army
In October, 1973, the Siri Singh Sahib received an urgent call from Europe that two men in the US Army, Privates James Broadwell and Richard Fresco, had taken Sikh

vows in the ashram, returned to their Army post in Germany with turbans on, and were immediately arrested and charged with noncompliance of Army dress regulations. They were offered an honorable discharge if they agreed not to force the issue, but they wanted to remain in the Army and refused to accept the discharge. They were given an immediate court-martial, were found guilty, and confined to the stockade where they were forcibly shaven and given a haircut. Upon their return to the United States, they again were held down and forcibly shaven in the Baltimore airport bathroom.

The people of Sikh Dharma felt shocked and betrayed by the actions of the United States Army. Every ashram throughout the Western Hemisphere began a letter campaign on behalf of the two soldiers. Gurdwaras and Sikh organizations in India and all over the world joined the Americans in the fight for religious freedom. Gurujot Singh went to Fort Riley, Kansas, where the soldiers were being held and presented himself as their Minister. The ACLU took up the case, and brought charges of abuse and civil rights violations against the Army. After a few days, a Federal Judge granted a temporary injunction protecting the men from further abuse and allowed them to wear their turbans in prison. The ashram in Kansas City received permission to hold Gurdwara services and yoga classes in prison for the soldiers.

Soon after this incident, Private Walter Scott and Navy man Ronald C. Sherwood also took Sikh vows and began wearing turbans in violation of the military dress code. They were also quickly court-martialed. After many months of persistent effort by Sikhs all over the world, on January 7, 1974, a US Army judge reversed the decision of the Army and declared the men not guilty of insubordination for wearing a turban, long hair, and beard while serving in the US Armed Forces. As a result, "A Sikh who is declared to be in good standing by his local Minister may be allowed to deviate from the Army dress code, by wearing beard, hair, turban, special underwear, comb, and a symbolic replica of a kirpan."[20]

Hari Nam Singh Elliot was the first American to join the Army as a practicing Sikh with a turban and full, uncut hair. He said, "Everyone I have met in the Army has shown a great deal of curiosity and disbelief."

Since that time, many Sikhs have served in the US Armed Forces, distinguishing themselves and honoring their country by their exemplary performance. The dress code exception was later overturned in 1981, and is currently still under appeal.

India Visits the West

Nineteen seventy-four marked the 100-year anniversary of the Singh Sabha movement in India and in honor of this, the Siri Guru Singh Sabha Shatabdhi Committee was touring the world, visiting and inspiring the sangats. Sardar Hukam Singh, President of the Siri Guru Singh Sabha Shatabdhi Committee; Sardar Gurucharan Singh Tohra, President of the S.G.P.C.; Giani Mahinder Singh, Secretary of the S.G.P.C.; and Sardar Surjit Singh Barnala, General Secretary of the Shiromani Akali Dal; left India on June 14 to begin a tour that was destined to inspire hundreds of thousands of Sikhs who had settled in the West. This visit would no doubt also affect their own perception of what was happening in the West as they saw for themselves a renaissance of Sikh Dharma in full bloom at the hands of and in the hearts of the western Sikhs.

This was the first time that Sikh leaders had left India on a mission such as this. Their visit had many aspects to it, but foremost was to meet and know the people who were leading the various sangats around the world and to understand the problems they faced. They were eager to meet the American Sikhs and understand how they had evolved to the position that they now held within the Panth. They wanted to know their background, their motivation, and to see how the Sikh way of life had blended in with American society.

This distinguished group first landed in New York City, and was greeted by the many Sikh sangats of that area. Here they met the new western-born Sikhs for the first time. Sardar Surjit Singh Barnala took time from his very busy schedule to stay at the Guru Ram Das Ashram in Brooklyn and participate in morning sadhana.

The weary Sardarjis arrived in Albuquerque, New Mexico in high spirits. The Summer Solstice Sadhana was taking place, and the airport reception was grand in scope and character. A Panj Piare dressed in full regalia greeted them with a five-sword salute as they walked off the airplane and into the terminal. About 100 small children sang to them the words of Guru Nanak, and the rest of the congregation cried out "Bole so Nihal!" over and over again.

Summer Solstice Sadhana was in process so this distinguished group traveled to the Solstice site and enjoyed several days with a sangat of over 1,000 people. They were excited by the devotion and dynamic energy they saw in the people of the camp. They remarked that the spirit shown by the sangat was like a return to the days of Guru Gobind Singh. The sangat in return was deeply honored and inspired by the visit of these esteemed guests. The Siri Guru Singh Sabha Shatabdhi Committee served the sangat as Punj Piare for the Amrit Parchar, and over 100 people partook of Amrit that day.

After Solstice, the Siri Singh Sahib and a kirtan jatha accompanied the Shatabdhi Committee to Canada to visit the sangats there. Here the Sikh leaders saw firsthand a source of tension between American and Indian Sikhs. They discovered that many of the Indian immigrants had shaved their beards and discarded their turbans. Their children were calling gurdwara a "church," and the *Siri Guru Granth Sahib* a "bible," and in this way, dissolving the unique form and nature of the Sikhs. At one gurdwara, the American jatha refused to enter and play kirtan until all the people in the sangat covered their heads. The Shatabdhi Committee stood firm with the Americans on this issue, and they waited at the door with the American jatha.

In an open letter to the sangat dated July 18, 1974, Sardar Hukam Singh and Sardar Gurucharan Singh Tohra wrote: "On the eve of our departure we wish to explain the purpose of our visit. The Shiromani Gurdwara Parbandhak Committee—Amritsar, had constituted a special committee to celebrate the Singh Sabha Centenary. The objectives were to re-emphasize the basic tenets of the Sikh Dharma, to start a campaign to recapture the dwindling moral values, and to stress the importance and essential necessity of the disciplines as enforced by Guru Gobind Singh Ji. The Singh Sabha Shatabdhi Committee carried on its work for the last 15 months in India. During this period, visits by two batches of the Canadian and American Sikhs evoked interest and even curiosity among the Sikhs in North India. Their firm conviction in the faith, the actual adoption of the Sikh way of life, and the strict observance of disciplines by these Canadian and American young boys and girls put to shame some young Sikhs who had deviated from the Sikh way of life. The S.G.P.C. appreciated the work done by 3HO and the Akal Takht decorated their leader as Siri Singh Sahib Harbhajan Singh Yogi recognizing him as head of the Sikh Dharma mission in the Western Hemisphere. We have observed during our tour that he had been doing this noble work admirably well." [21]

Yatras to India in 1974

In February, 1974, a group of western Sikhs returned to India and the blessed Harimandir Sahib. Here again, many western born Sikhs took Amrit and entered into the order of the Khalsa.

Accompanied by Sardar Gurucharan Singh Tohra, President of the S.G.P.C., the jatha toured the gurdwaras of Punjab giving Gurbani Kirtan programs and meeting with people. At Anandpur Sahib the ladies, all of whom were Khalsa and most of whom were ministers, petitioned to do seva in the gurdwara. This was traditionally an honor reserved only for men. S. Gurucharan Singh worked it out, and so it was that Bibiji Inderjit Kaur became the first woman in history to clean the weapons of Guru Gobind Singh Ji.

The Siri Singh Sahib arrived in New Delhi with his children, who traveled on to Mussoorie to attend school. Upon arriving in Amritsar, the Siri Singh Sahib was royally received at the airport by the S.G.P.C. and was able to spend a few precious days at the Harimandir Sahib.

He returned to Delhi to attend the World Conference on the Unity of Man sponsored by Sant Kirpal Singh of the Ruhani Satsang. This huge event was attended by top level religious, social, and political leaders from all over the world. The Siri Singh Sahib stayed in India for only seven days, and then flew on to London and Amsterdam to teach White Tantric Yoga in those cities.

In November, an American jatha again traveled to India to attend the 52nd All-India Sikh Educational Conference. Ram Das Singh accompanied the jatha, and his long and flowing beard was eyed with much respect. "It seems that after taking a look at Ram Das Singh's beard, those Indian gentlemen took a second look at their own. During the first day of the conference, as the Sikh jatha from America was just about to play kirtan, one of the organizers of the conference stood up boldly, firmly untying his rolled beard and pledged before the Guru and the sangat that from that day onward he would always take pride in a loose, flowing beard. More directors and leaders solemnly vowed before the Guru and the sangat that they would never tie their beards again, drink, or indulge in any practices detrimental to the Sikh way of life."[22]

The Siri Singh Sahib came from America and joined the group in Amritsar for the great occasion of Guru Ram Das's birthday. As Nirinjan Kaur writes: "The crowds of people at the Harimandir Sahib were tantamount to the numbers of people attending the Woodstock Festival in New York a few years ago!" As was the Siri Singh Sahib's practice, nearly every hour of the day and night was devoted to talking with people, sharing in their laughter, comforting their sorrows, assuring them that God and Guru are guiding and preparing everyone's destiny.

Since the Shatabdhi Committee had recently returned to India, they had informed the rest of the Sikh leadership about the rebirth of Sikh Dharma in the West. On the November 13, 1974, the Siri Singh Sahib was honored with the exalted title of "Bhai Sahib" at the Akal Takhat for his dedication to spreading the mission of the Gurus. Before thousands of people, the Siri Singh Sahib accepted the saropa, sword, and a beautifully engraved silver plate from the Jathedar of the Akal Takhat. Few Sikhs are given this honor and, like his grandfather before him, the Siri Singh Sahib accepted the prayers of the sangat with grace and humility.

When the jatha returned to New Delhi, the Siri Singh Sahib attended the Fifth World Religious Conference. He played an active role in this event in his continuing mission to unite the world's religions. The outcome of the conference was the establishment of the "World Parliament of Religions" and he was elected as its first Chairman.

Throughout India, the Siri Singh Sahib addressed the sangat on many occasions reminding them of their destiny and responsibilities as Khalsa. He chastised those Sikhs who had deviated from the Rehit of Guru Gobind Singh. "You are distinct, and that is the way you should look. Guru Gobind Singh has said it clearly:

> *Jab lag khaalsaa rahe niaaraa. Tab lag tej deeo mai saaraa. Jab eh gahai biparan kee reet. Mai naa karo in kee parteet.*

> *So long as Khalsa retains his distinct identity, I will give him my entire strength. But if he should take on a non-Sikh way of life, then I shall have confidence in him no more.*
>
> Guru Gobind Singh Ji; Sarab Loh Granth

"When you live a very distinct and disciplined life, Guru Gobind Singh promises that he will inject you with the entire cosmic power of radiance and spirit. So it is in your hands, there is no use in living half-minded. Value not social pressures, they have always been exerted on men of God."

After speaking at Bangla Sahib Gurdwara one day toward the end of the tour, the Siri Singh Sahib was making his way through the crowds to leave when suddenly a man charged at him with a sword held high over his head. Sardarni Guru Amrit Kaur, who had been a championship fencer in college, quickly moved in front of the Siri Singh Sahib and raised her forearm against the attacker, successfully blocking the sword blow that was aimed at the Siri Singh Sahib's head. Although she was cut on the arm she showed no concern for her own safety. Grabbing the man, she threw him aside. Together with Sat Peter Singh, they moved the Siri Singh Sahib to safety through the excited and agitated crowd. Meanwhile the Delhi police quickly mobilized and dealt with the attacker and his cohorts.

In the final press conference of the trip, the Siri Singh Sahib said, "Let not opposition stand in the way of our mission in life. In fact, welcome it, feel grateful for it, as it only makes us fight harder and faster in unity for a cause that will create peace and harmony. Spiritualism was hatched in the East, but as Guru Teg Bahadur meditated facing the West, and just as Guru Gobind Singh pointed to the West, there is now a stirring happening there. These young people have the insides of a saint, and the outsides of a soldier and they will not rest until they see the rightful destiny of joy and happiness shining on the faces of all their brothers and sisters. Behold their example!"

Notes

1. *Beads of Truth*, Sept. 1973
2. *Beads of Truth*, June 1973
3. Paul Singh Kaufman; *Beads of Truth*, June 1973
4. *Beads of Truth*, March 1973
5. *Beads of Truth*, June 1974,
6. Shakti Parwha Kaur; *Beads of Truth*, December 1972
7. *Beads of Truth*, March 1973
8. Gurubanda Singh; *Beads of Truth* 1976
9. *Beads of Truth* 1973
10. Gurucharan Kaur; *Beads of Truth*, June 1973
11. *Beads of Truth*, Fall 1975
12. *Beads of Truth*, Sept. 1973
13. S. Premka Kaur; *Beads of Truth*, Sept. 1974
14. Krishna Kaur; *Beads of Truth*, Winter 1973
15. Gurujot Kaur; *Sikh Dharma Brotherhood Magazine,* March 1973
16. *Beads of Truth*, Spring 1974
17. Yogi Bhajan
18. In yogic terminology, the left and right nostrils are energy channels, or nadis, known as the ida and pingala respectively
19. Yogi Bhajan: *Sikh Dharma Brotherhood Magazine,* Baisakhi 1976
20. *Army Command Policy & Procedure, Beads of Truth,* June 1974
21. *Beads of Truth*, Sept. 1974
22. Nirinjan Kaur; *Beads of Truth*, Spring 1975

The Spark
by S.S. Gurutej Singh Khalsa

There was a time, some may remember,
When the spirit in us was like an ember
And at that time, some may recall,
We began to rise and answer the call.

There was a point, some began to know,
That the ember in us had begun to glow.
It spread through us, to our delight,
For that glowing ember was Guru's Light.

For twenty-five years, some might suggest,
The ember was fanned by challenge and test;
And fueled by sacrifice, surrender and pain
It has caught the heart and burst into flame!

The Children of the Cusp, we might be called,
Have started a fire that can't be controlled.
Blown from the Heavens, by the Winds of Change,
The Consciousness of Man it will rearrange.

But let us remember, that once we were dark,
Then hammer and chisel ignited that spark,
And that humble artist, who put blade to stone,
Walks through the flames to sleep in the Dome.

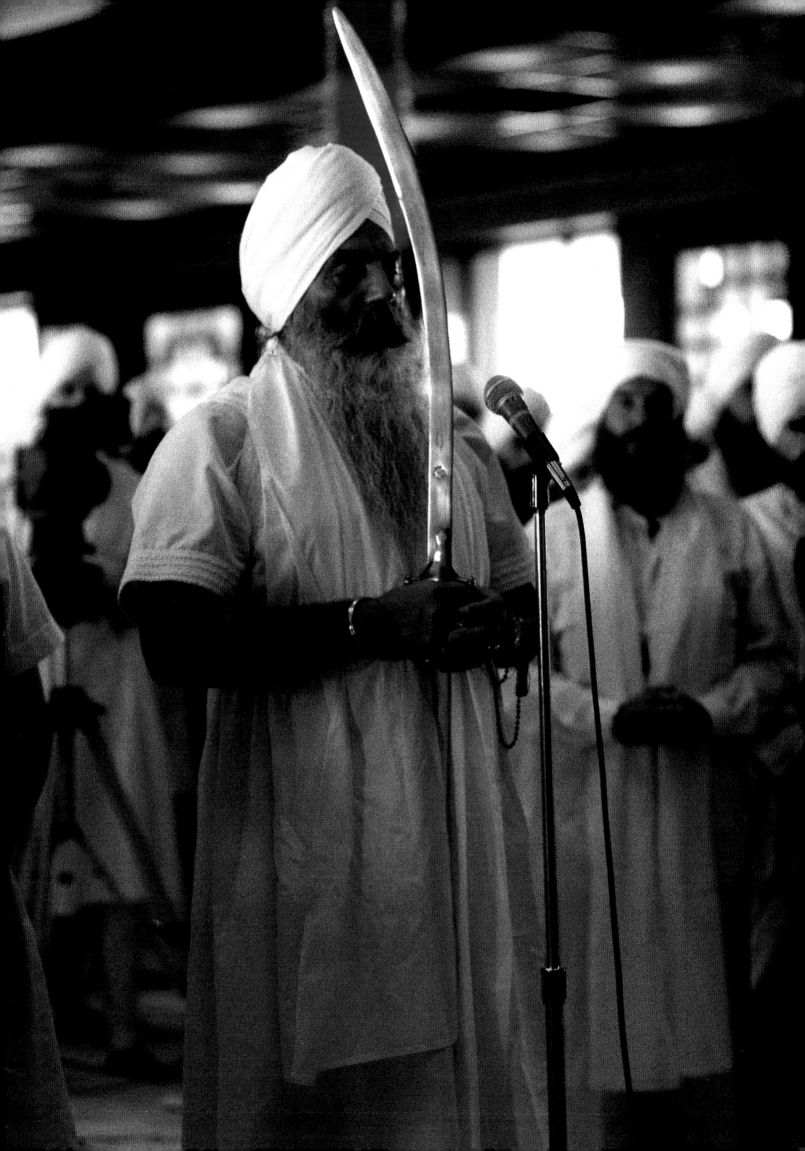

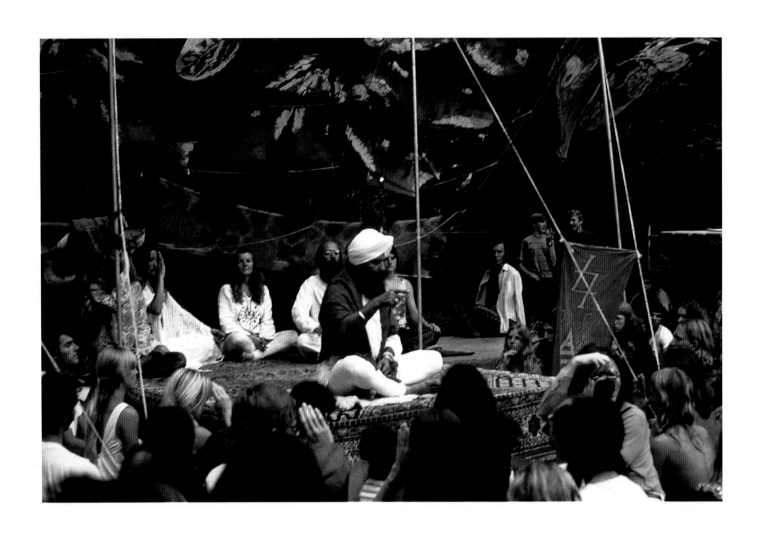

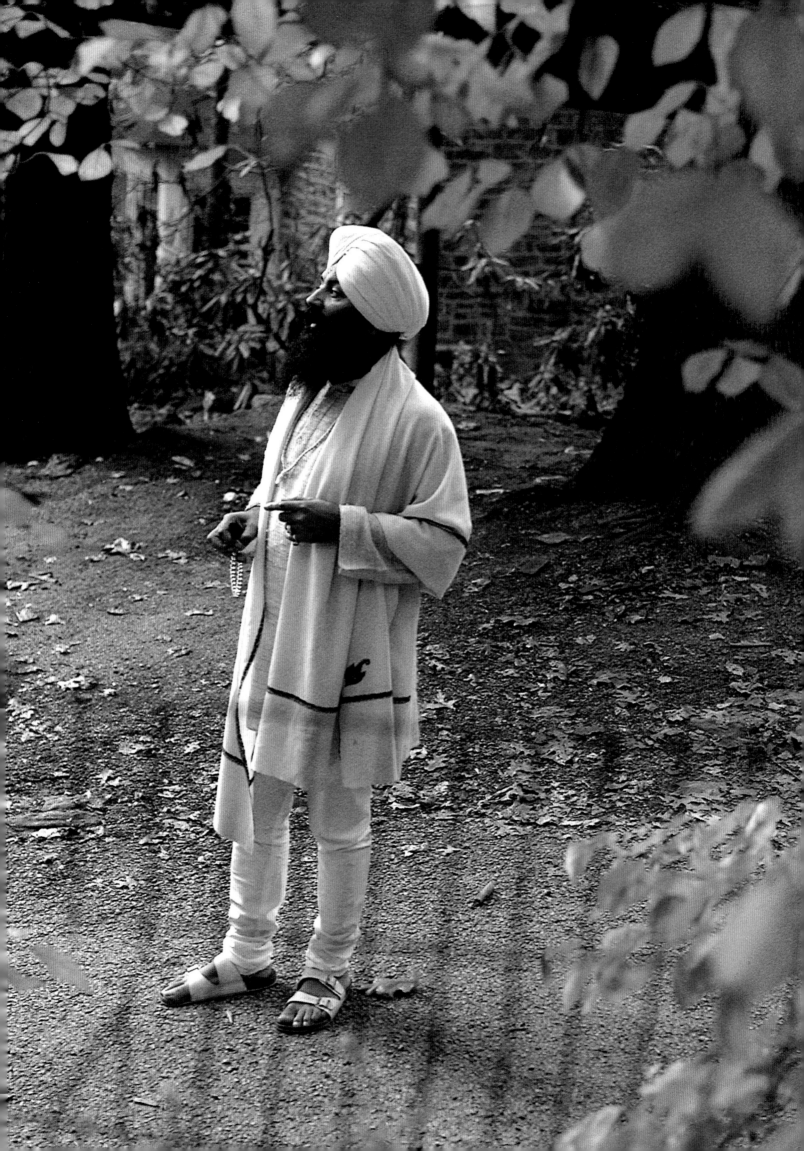

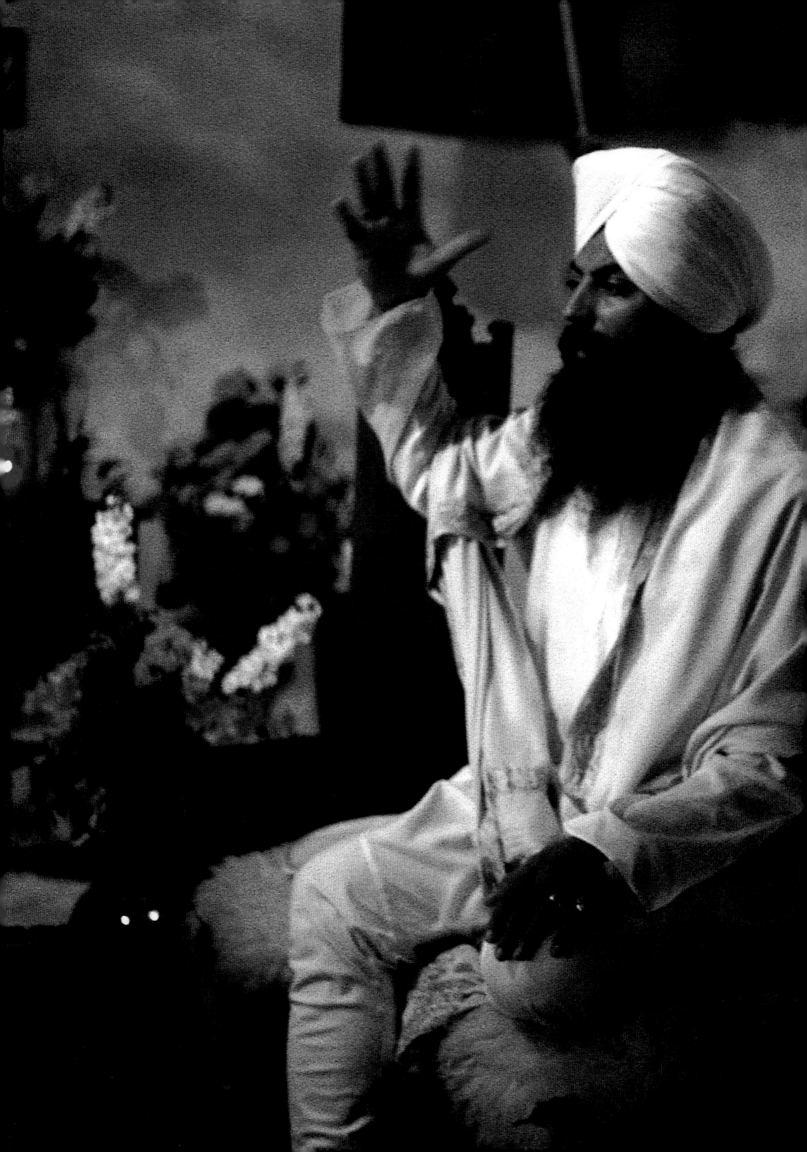

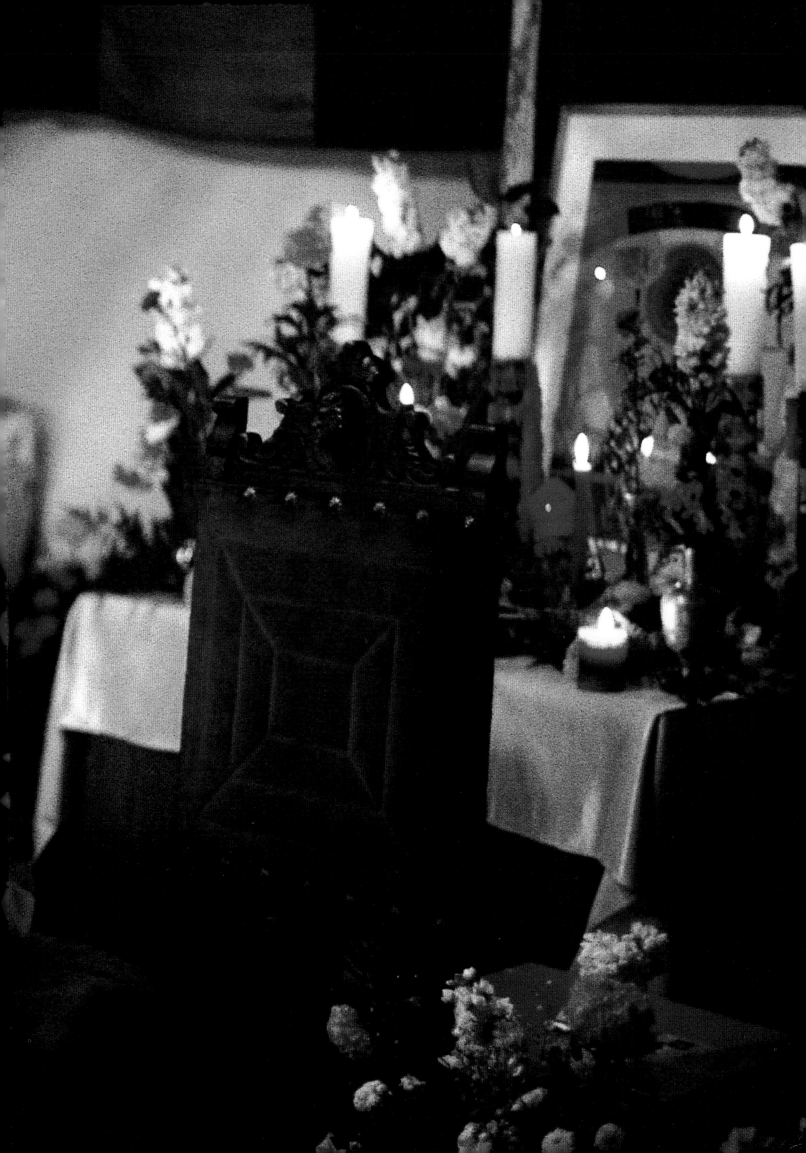

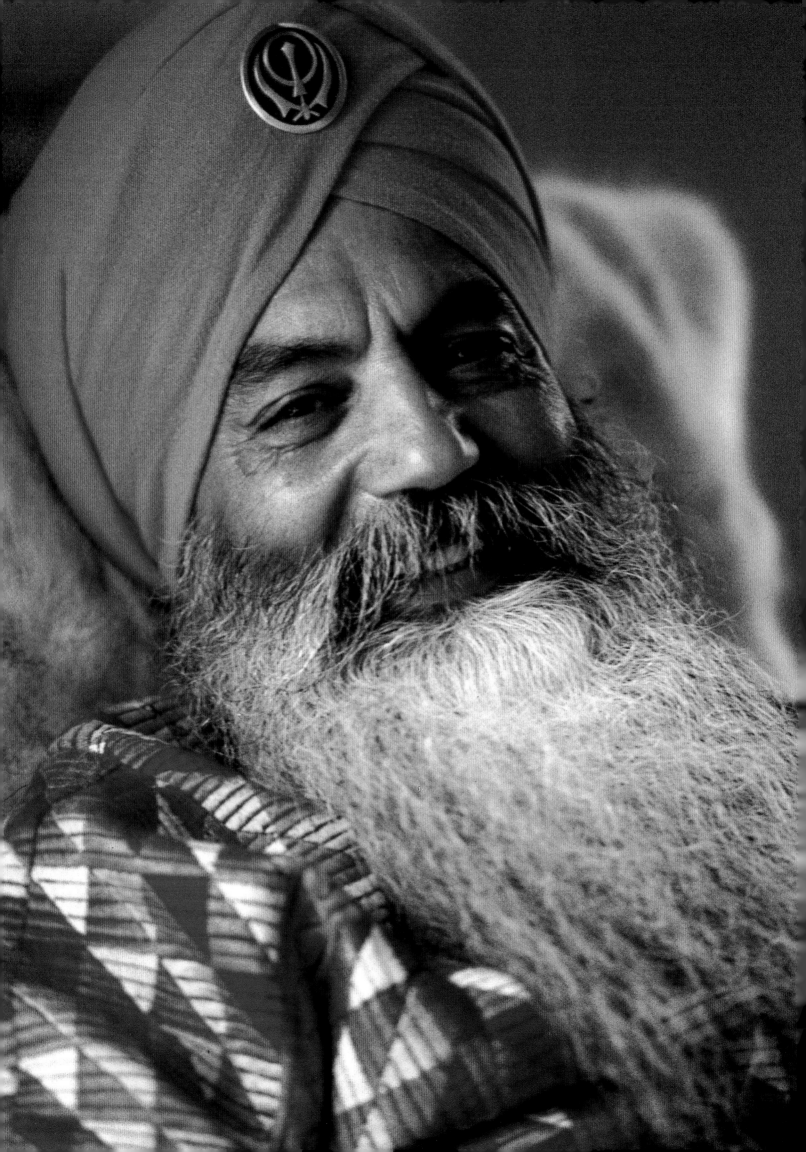

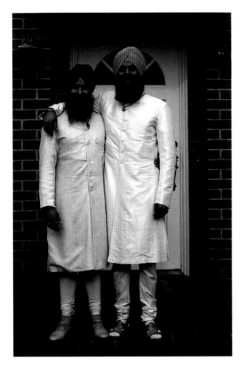
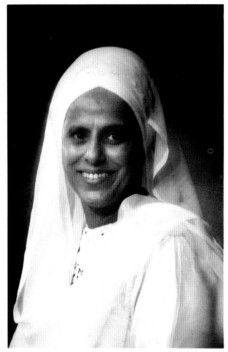
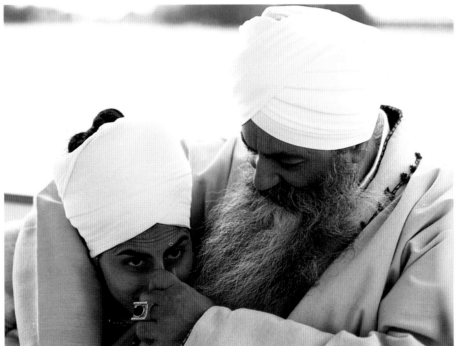

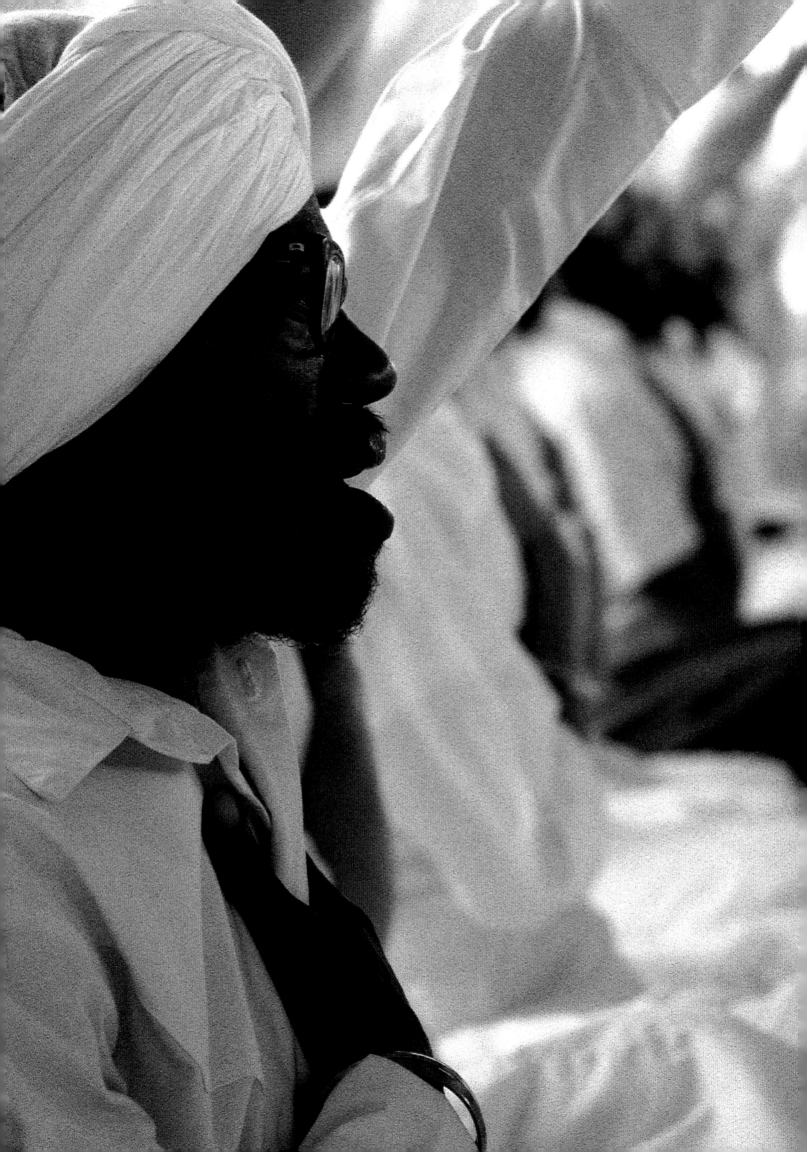

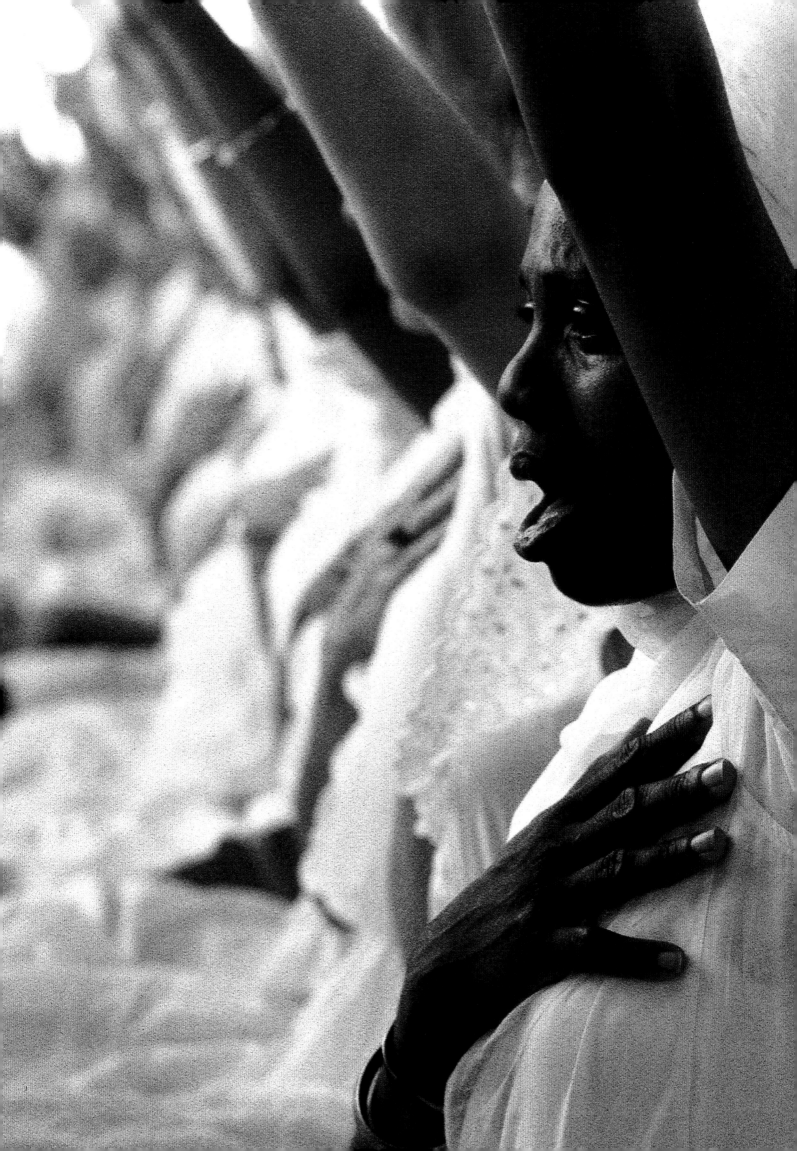

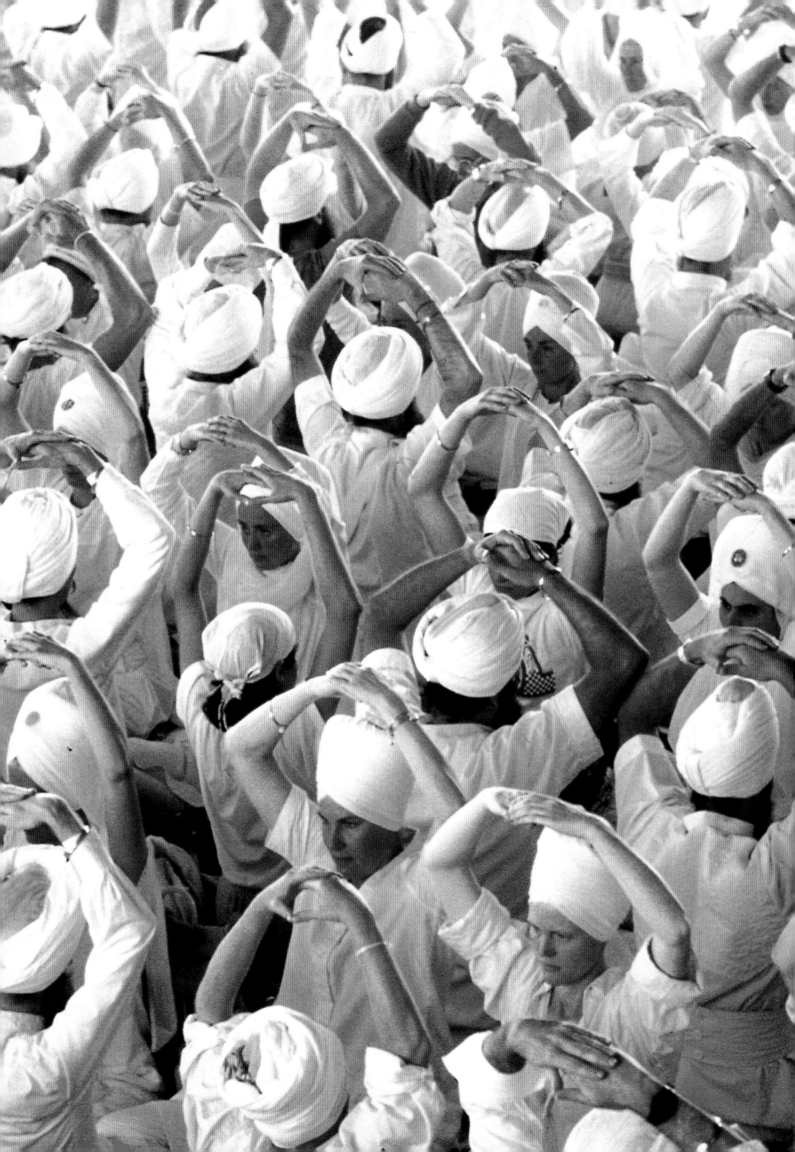

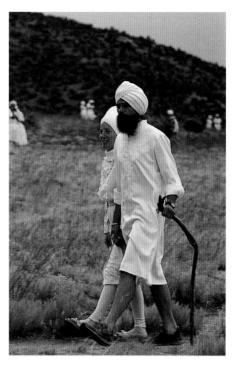

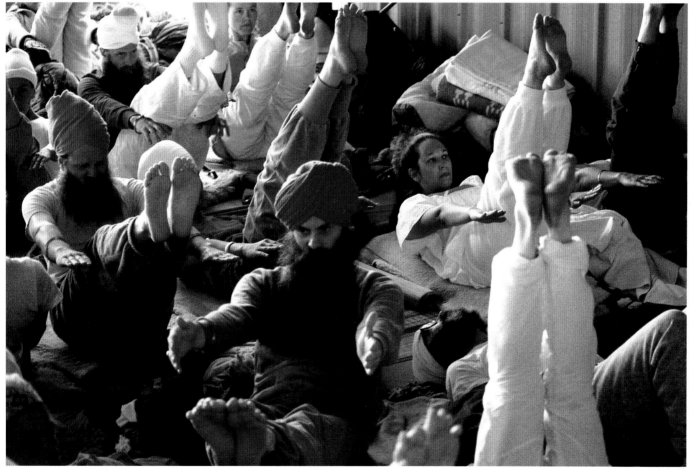

63

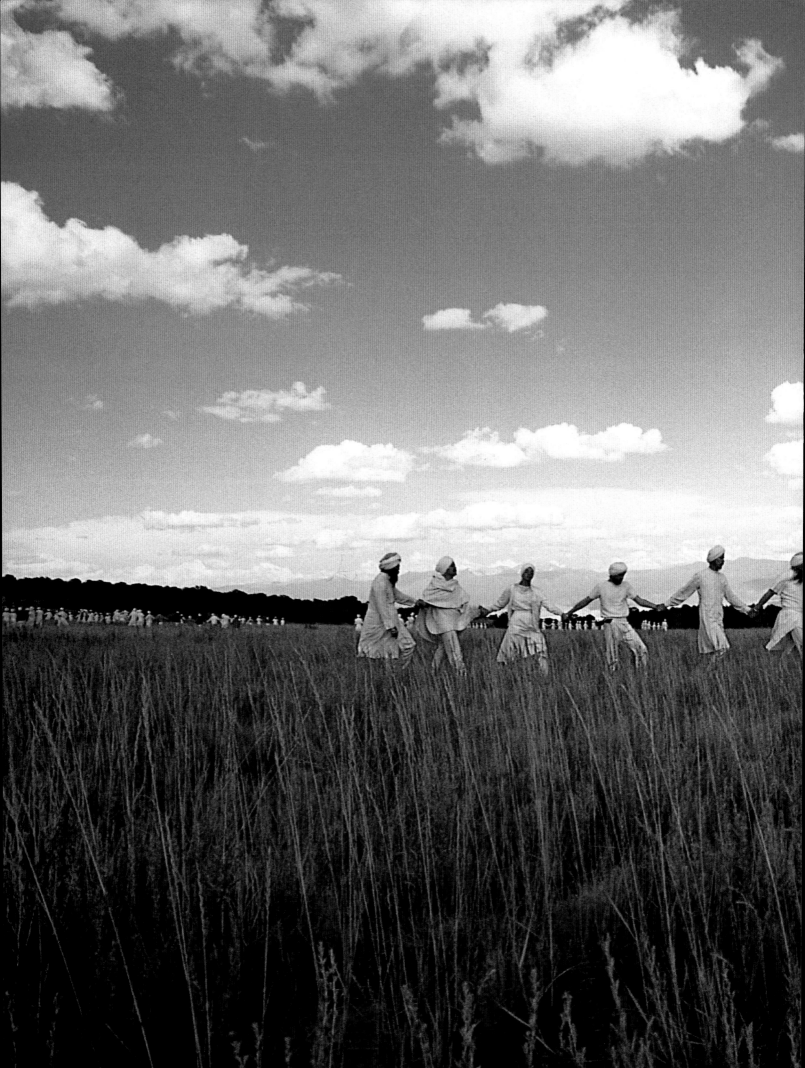

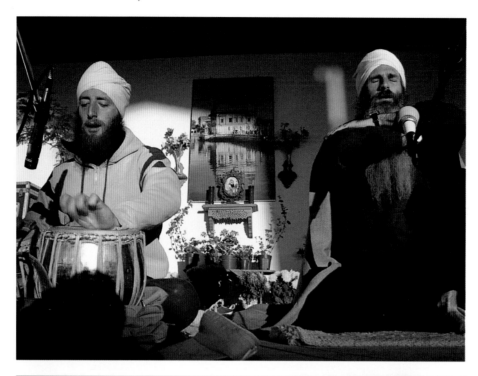

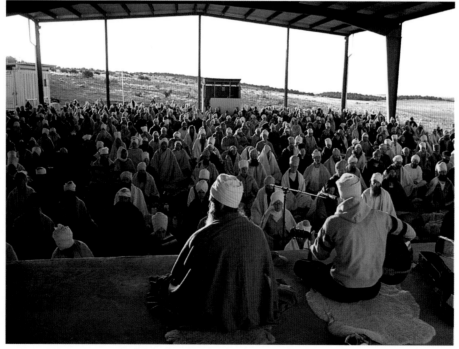

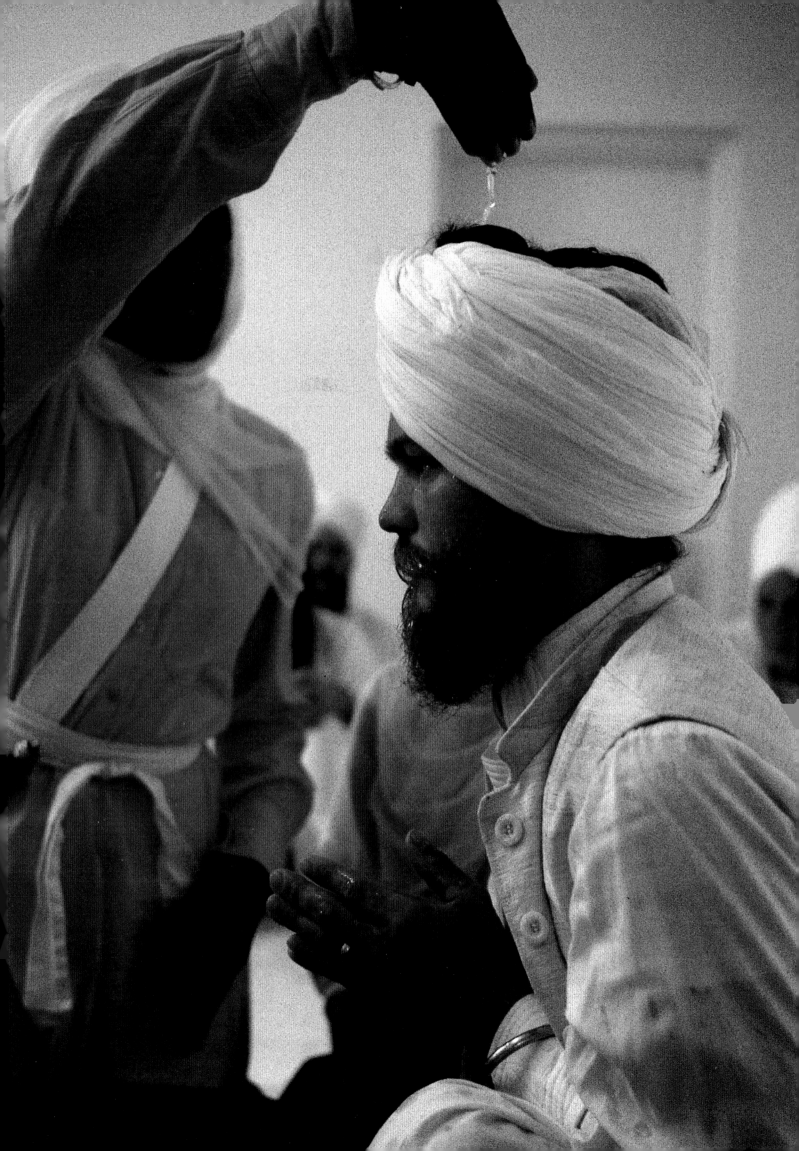

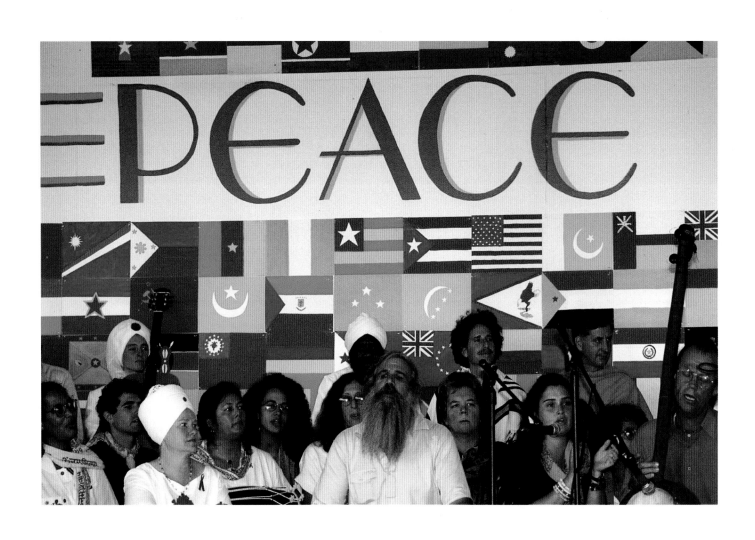

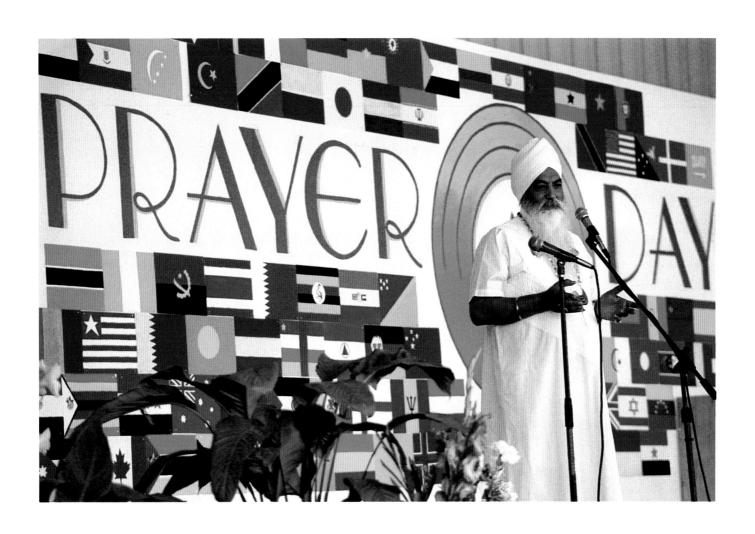

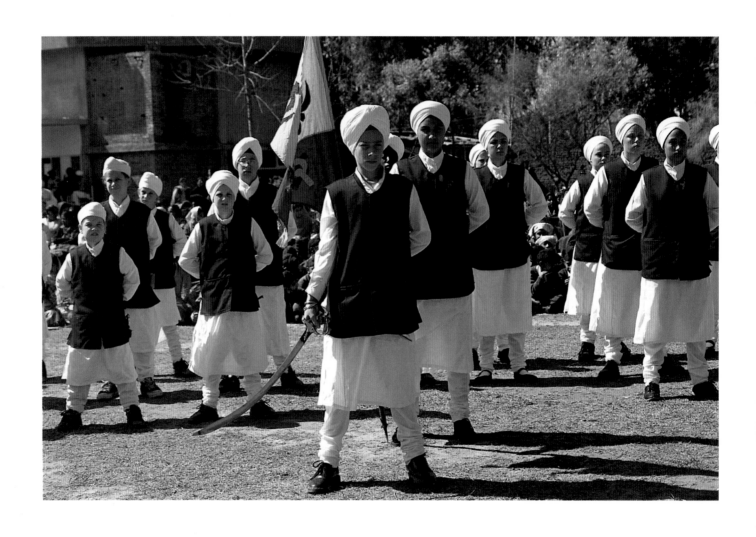

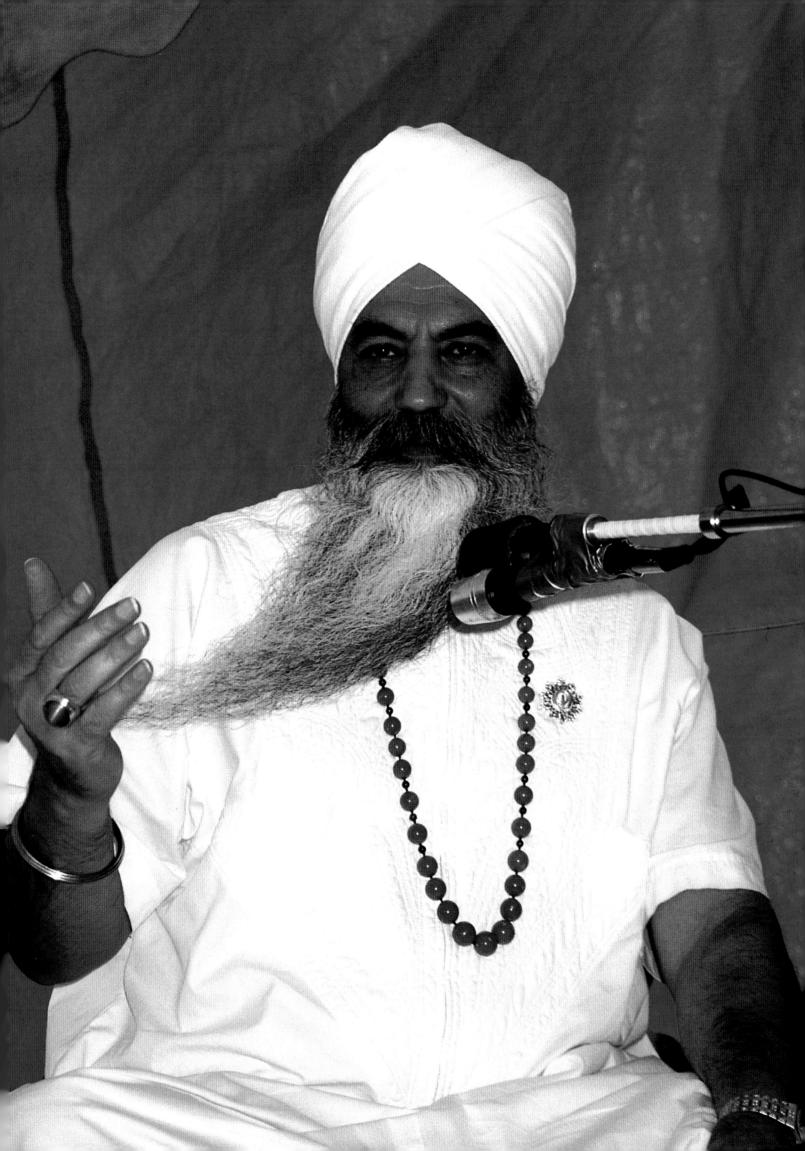

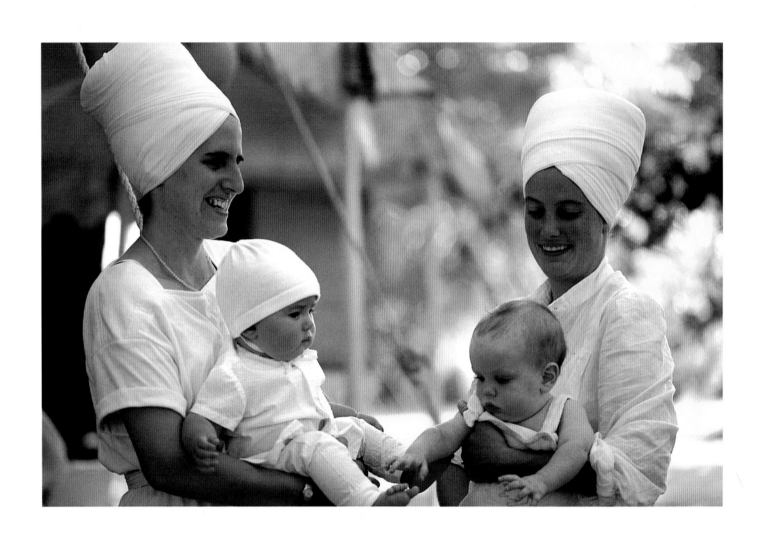

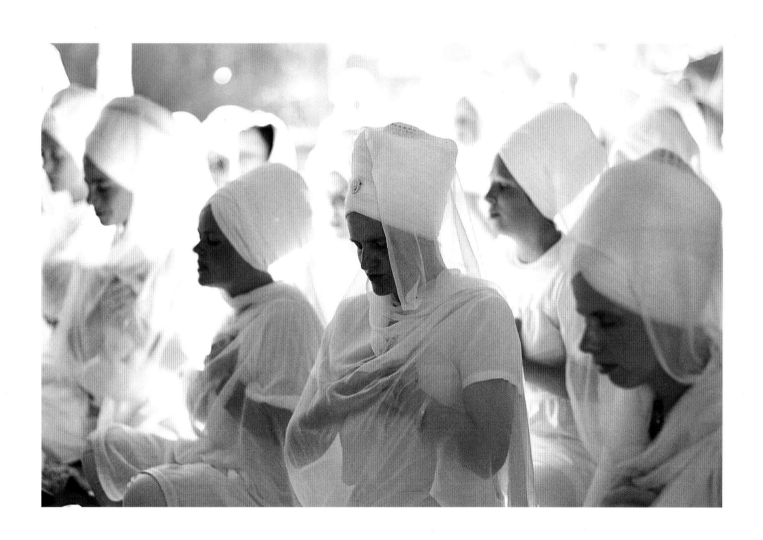

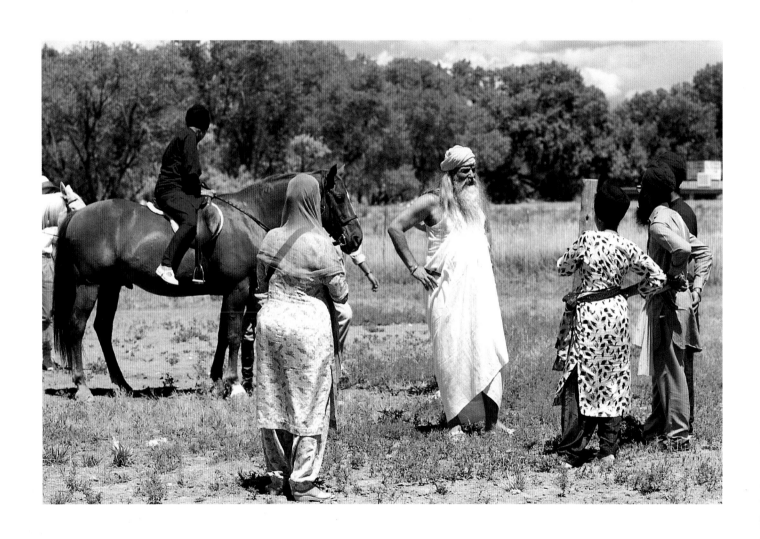

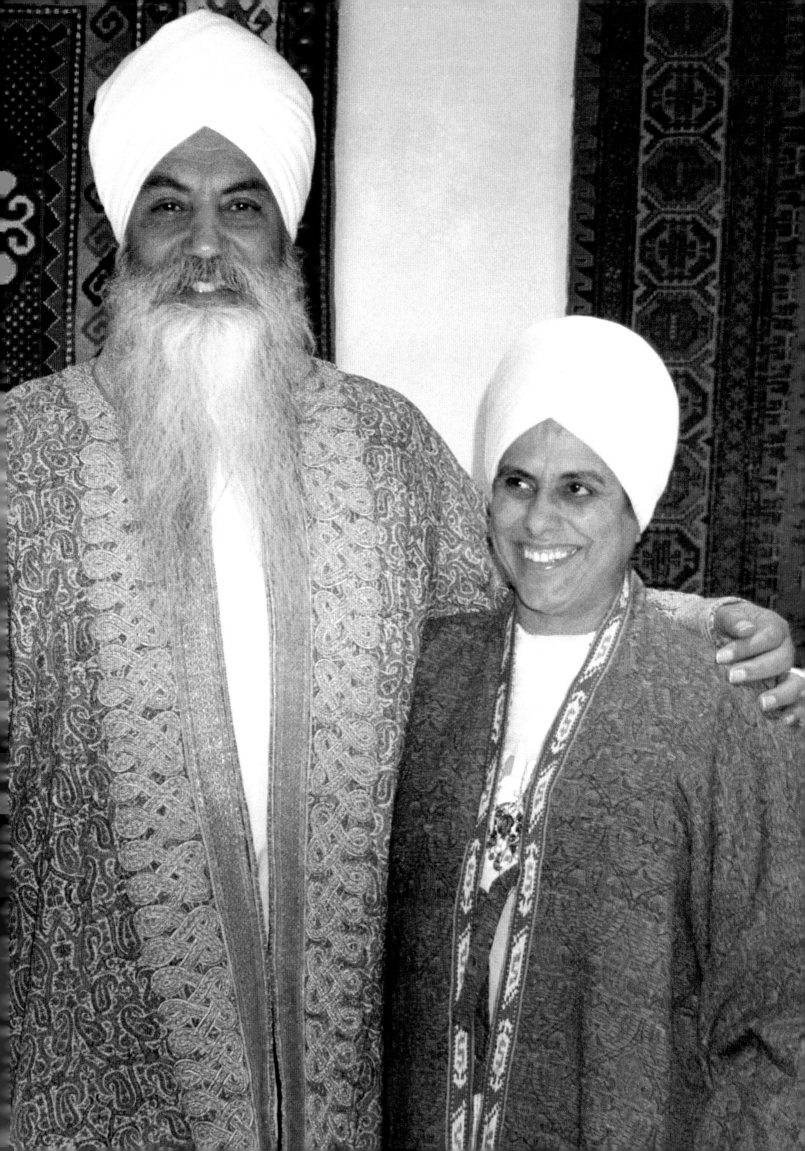

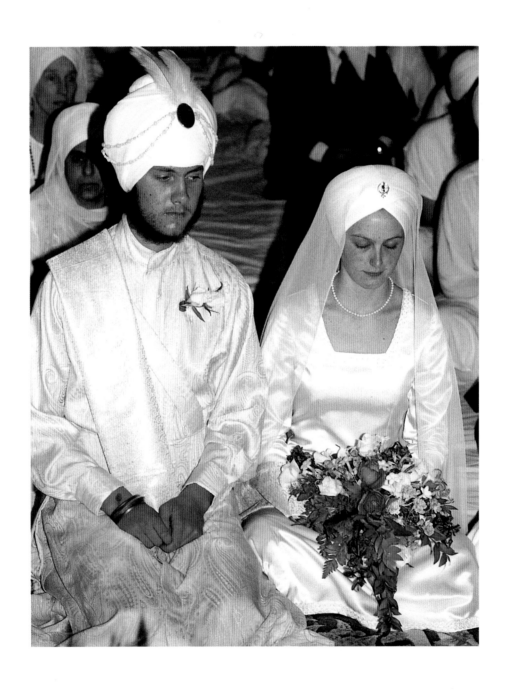

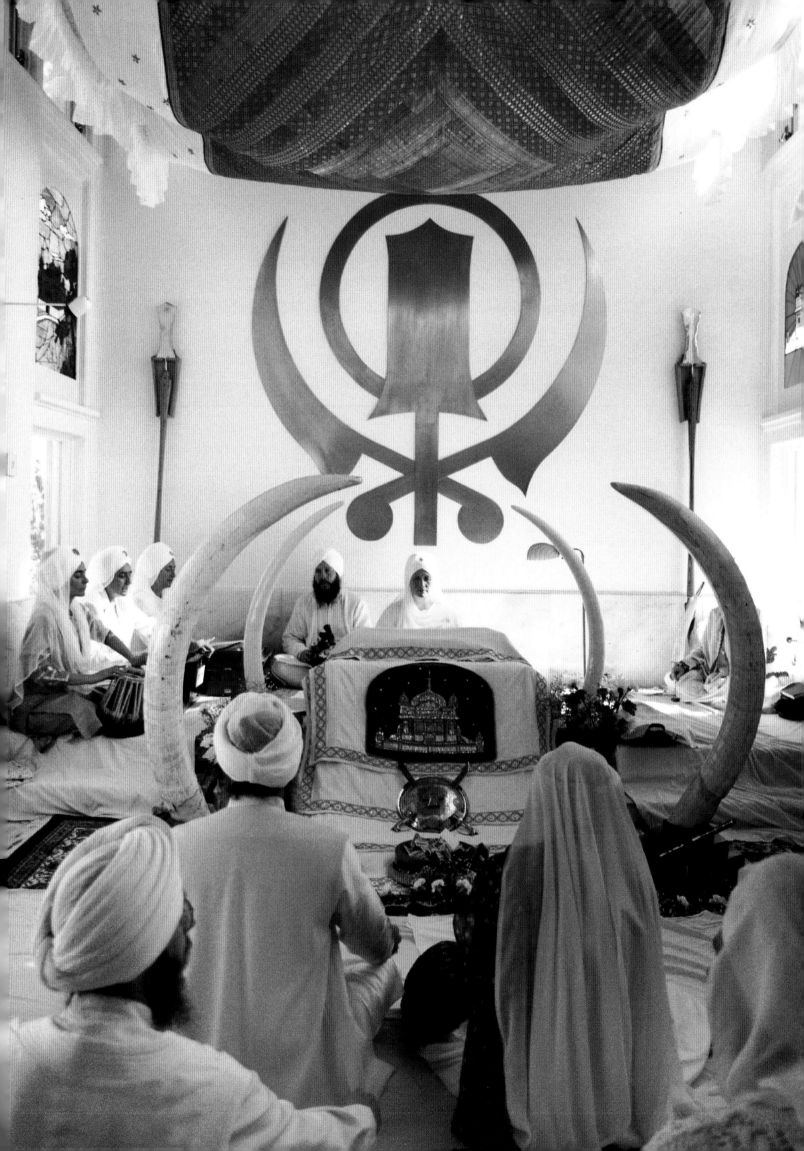

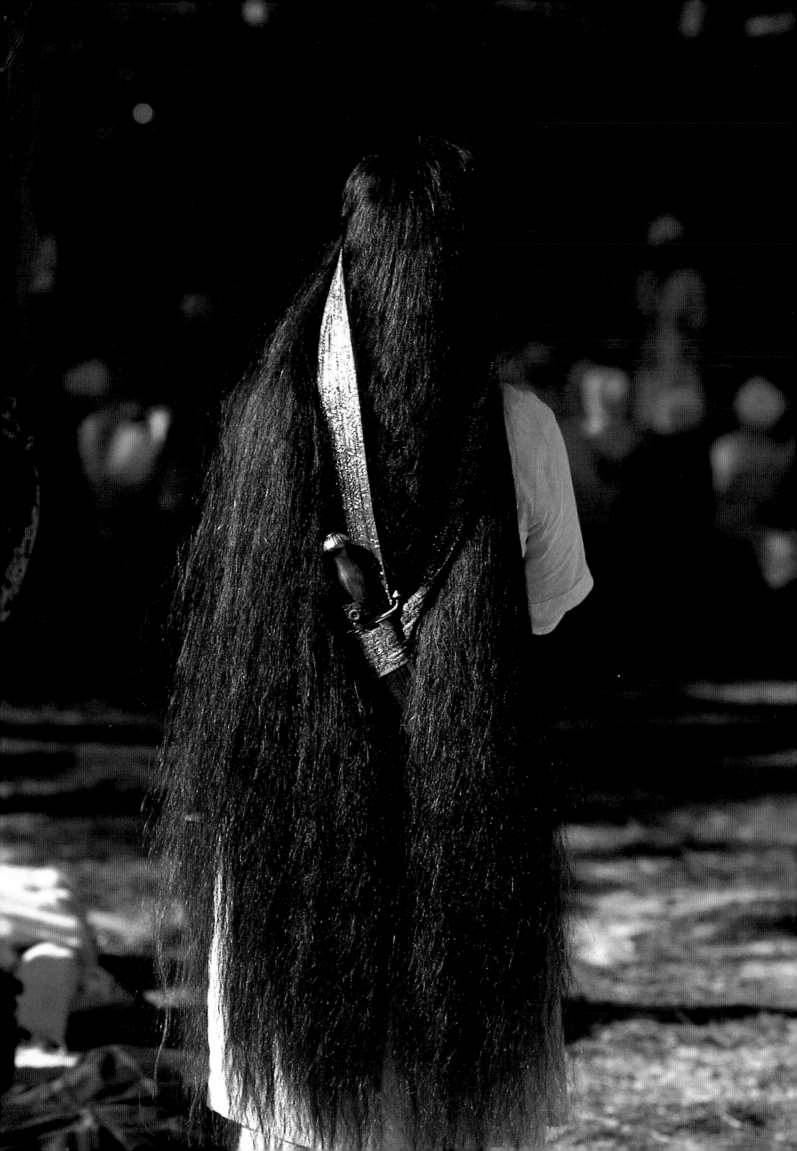

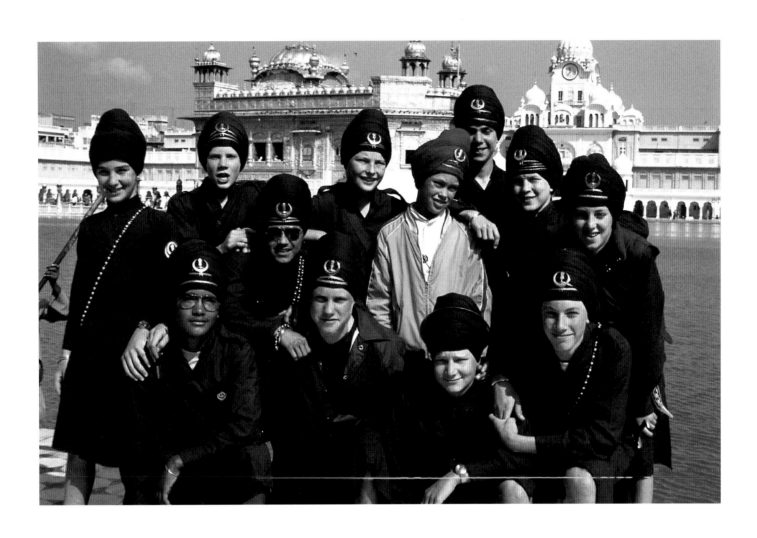

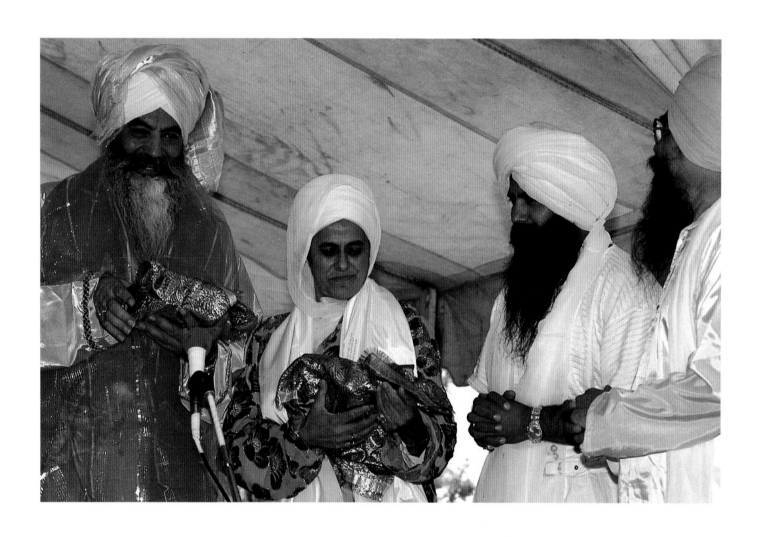

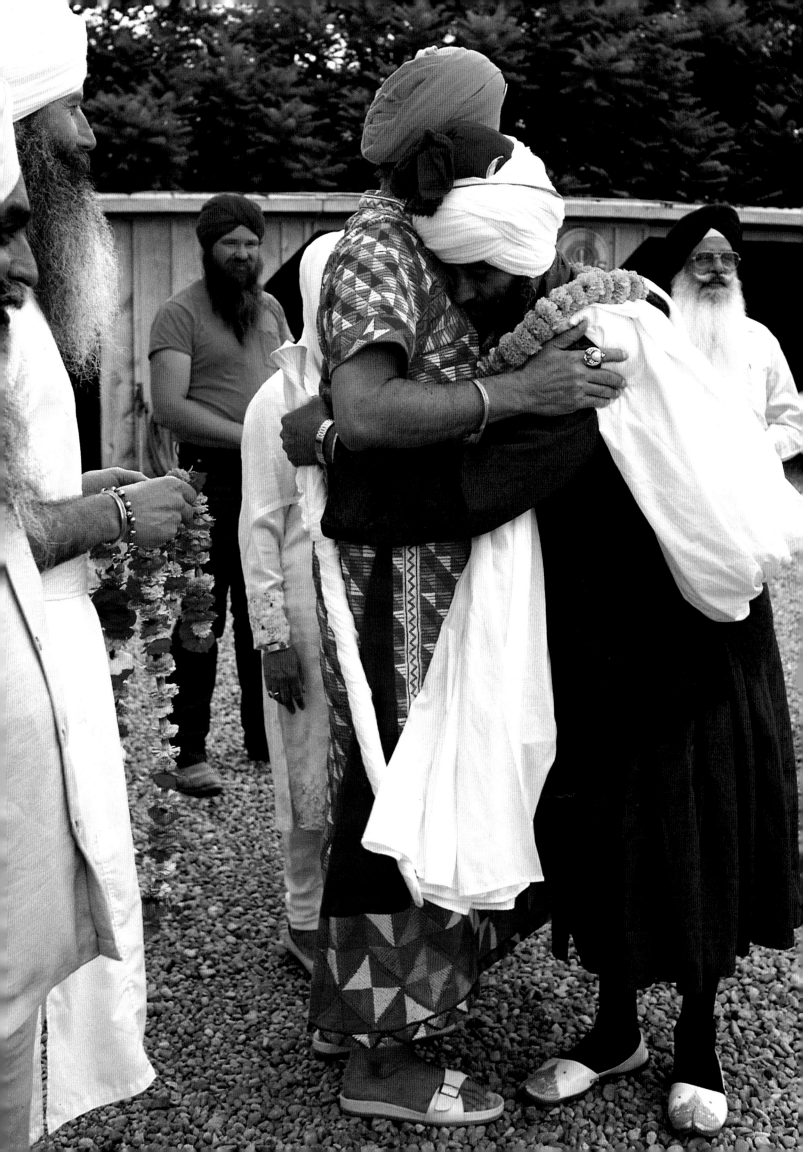

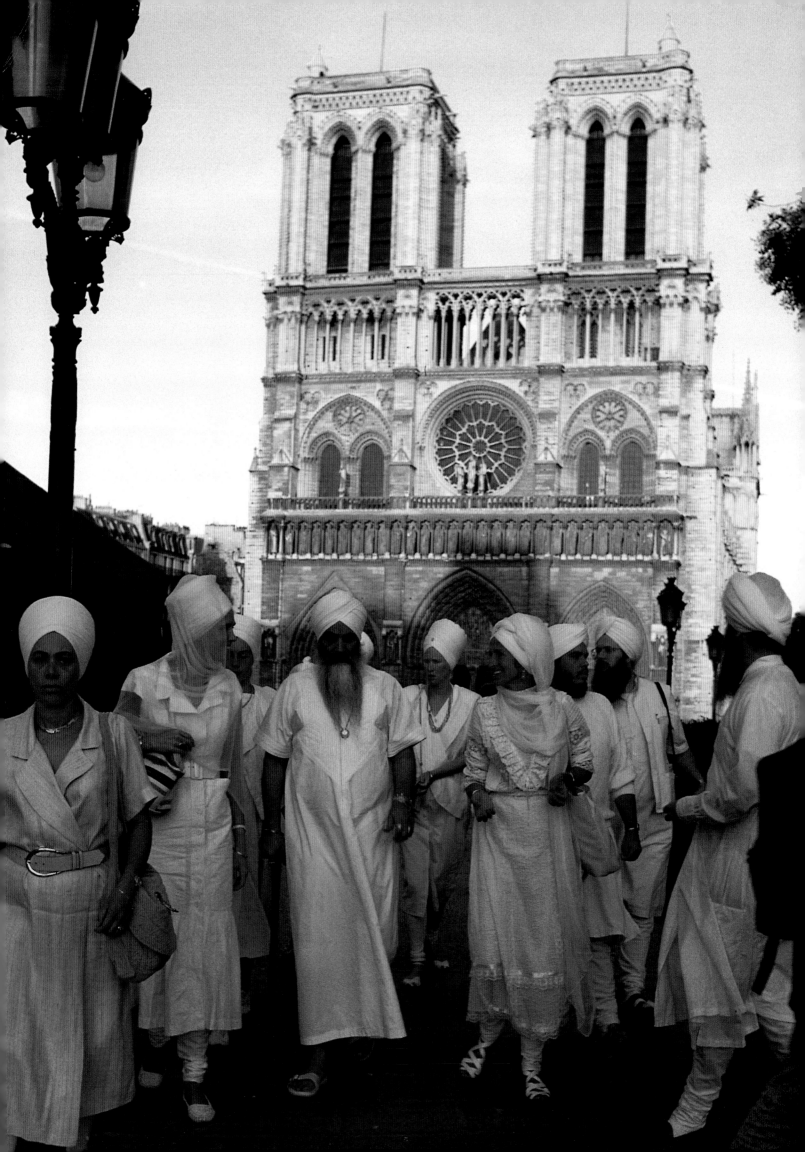

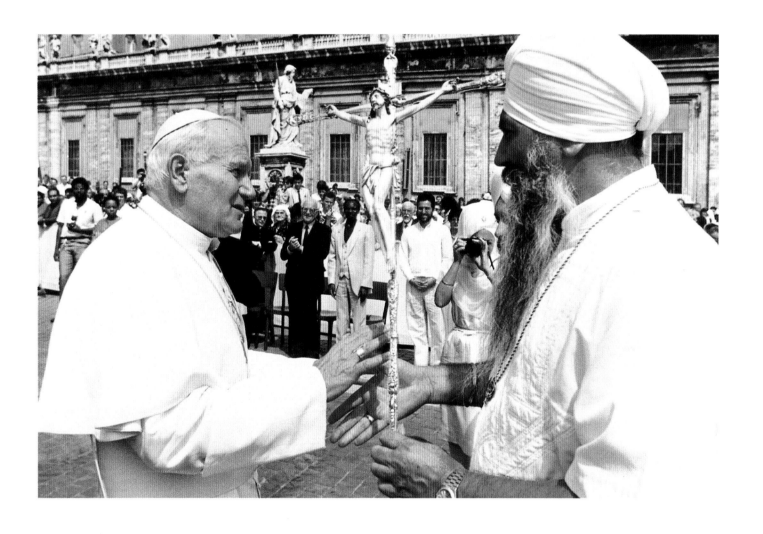

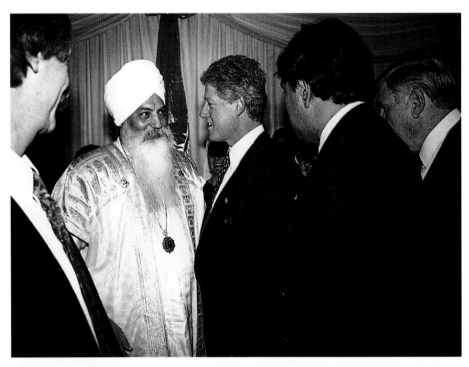

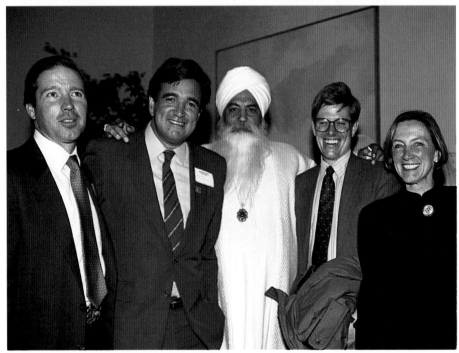

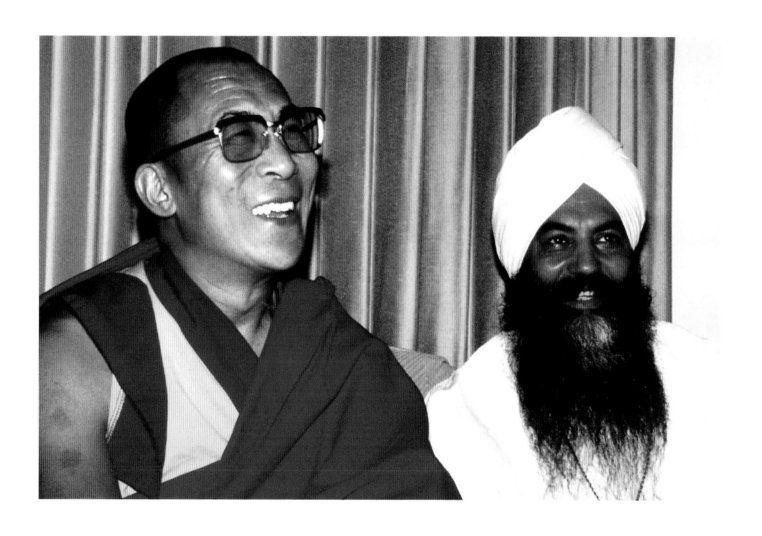

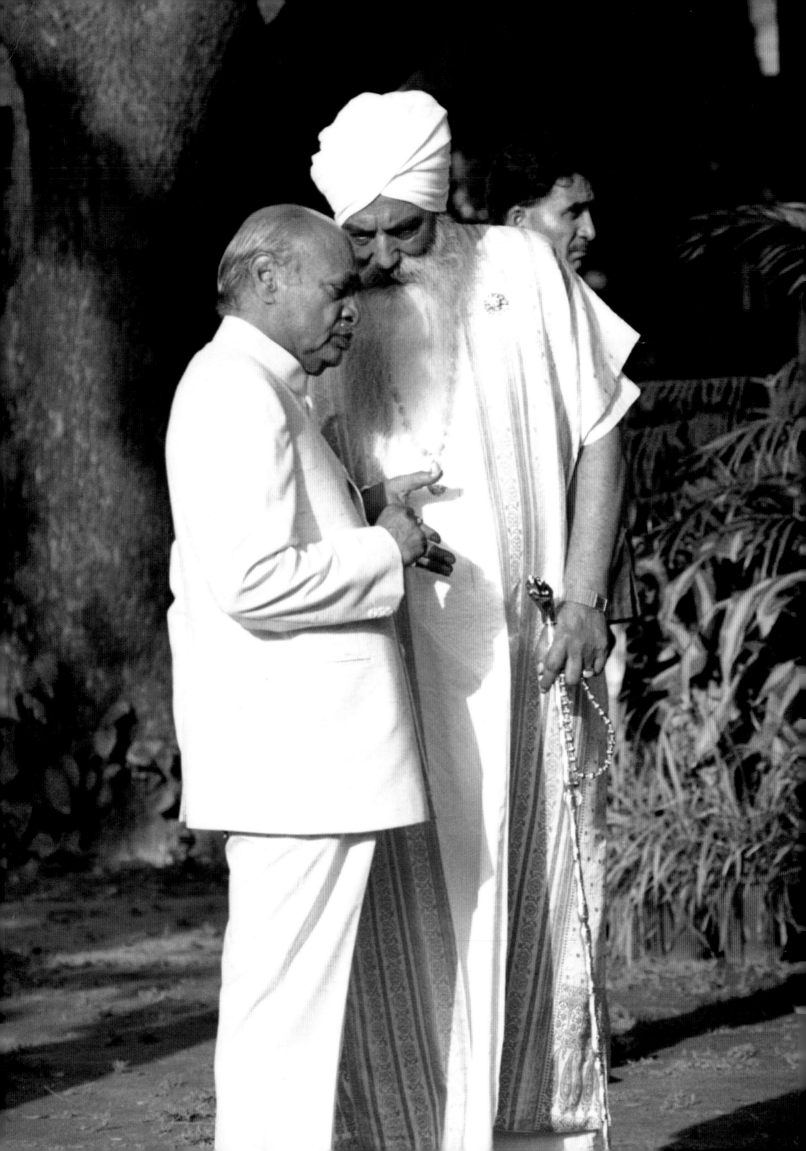

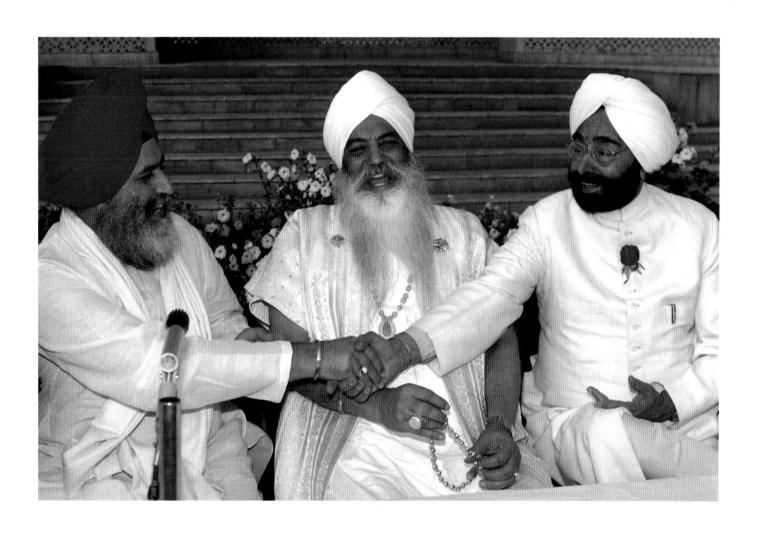

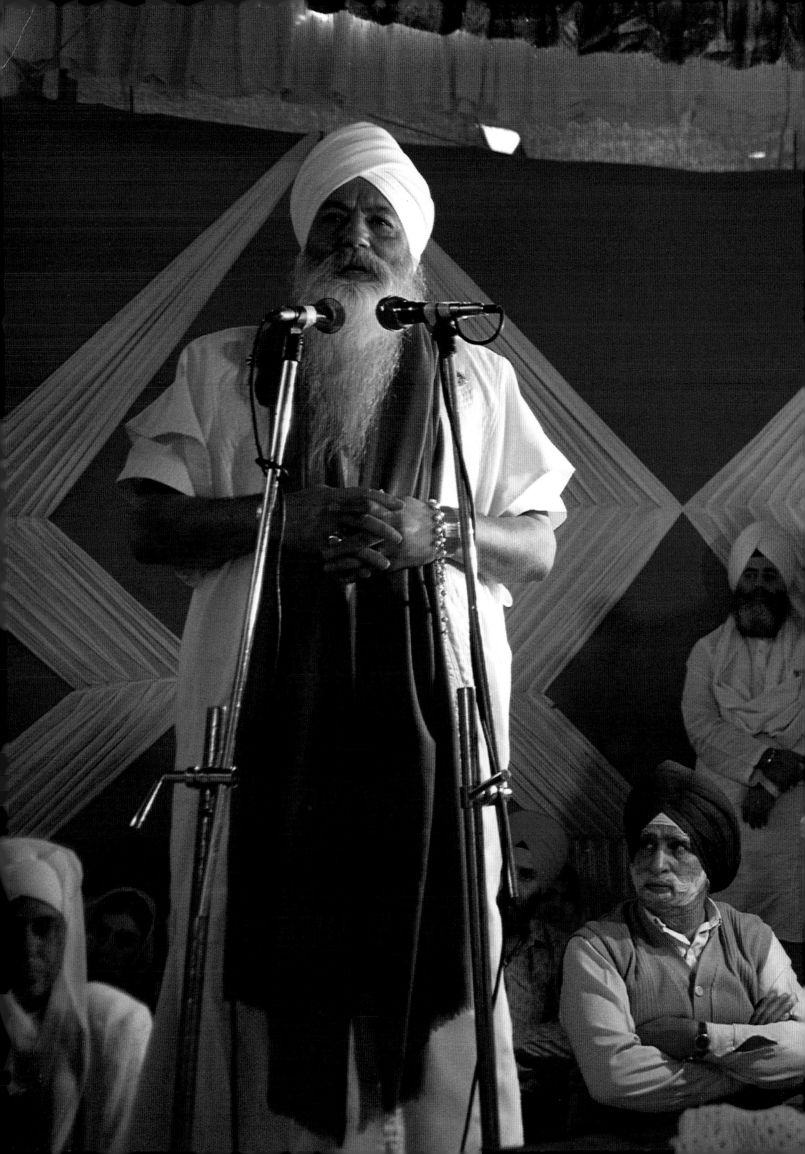

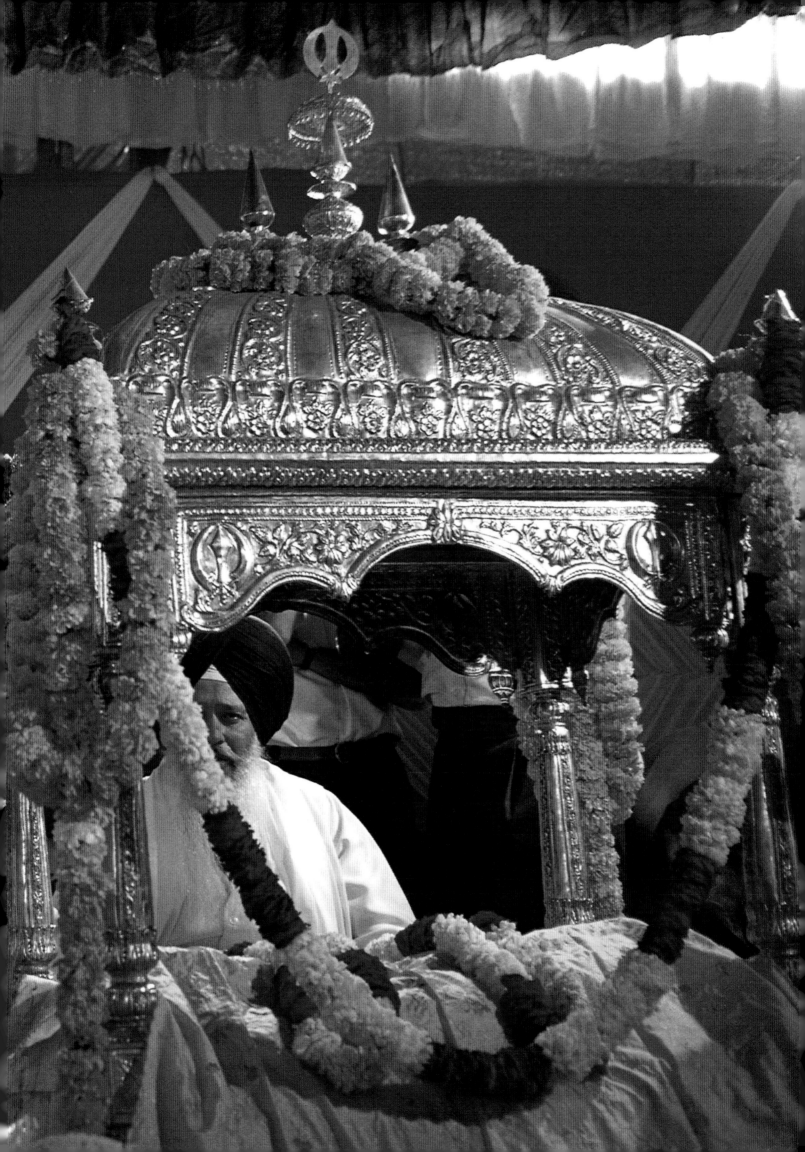

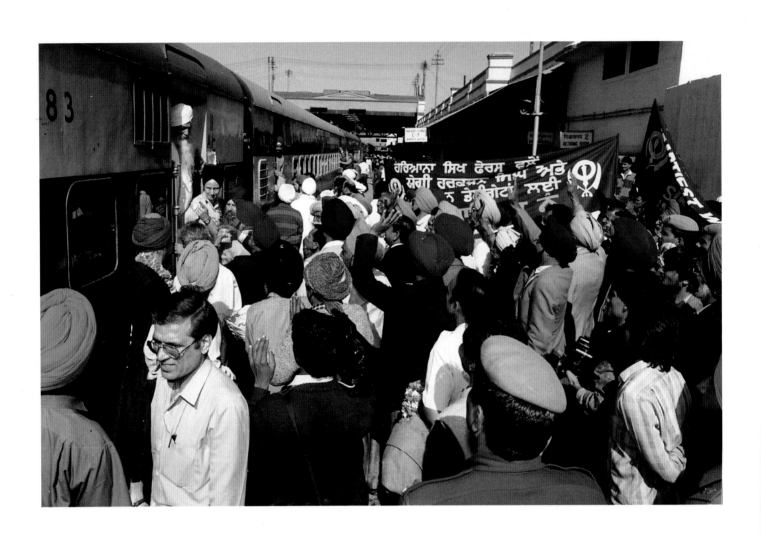

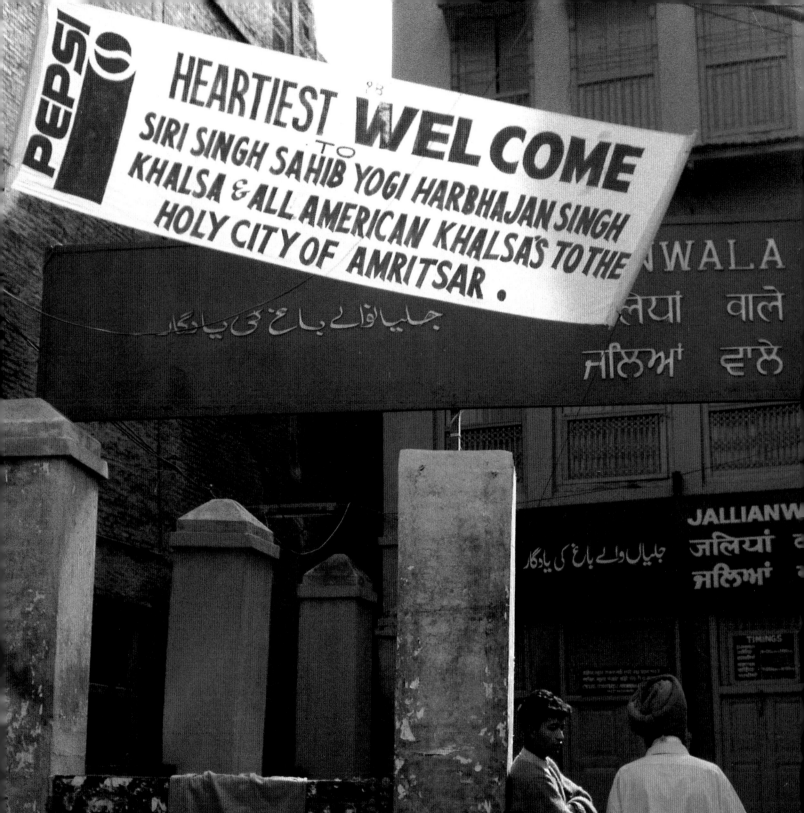

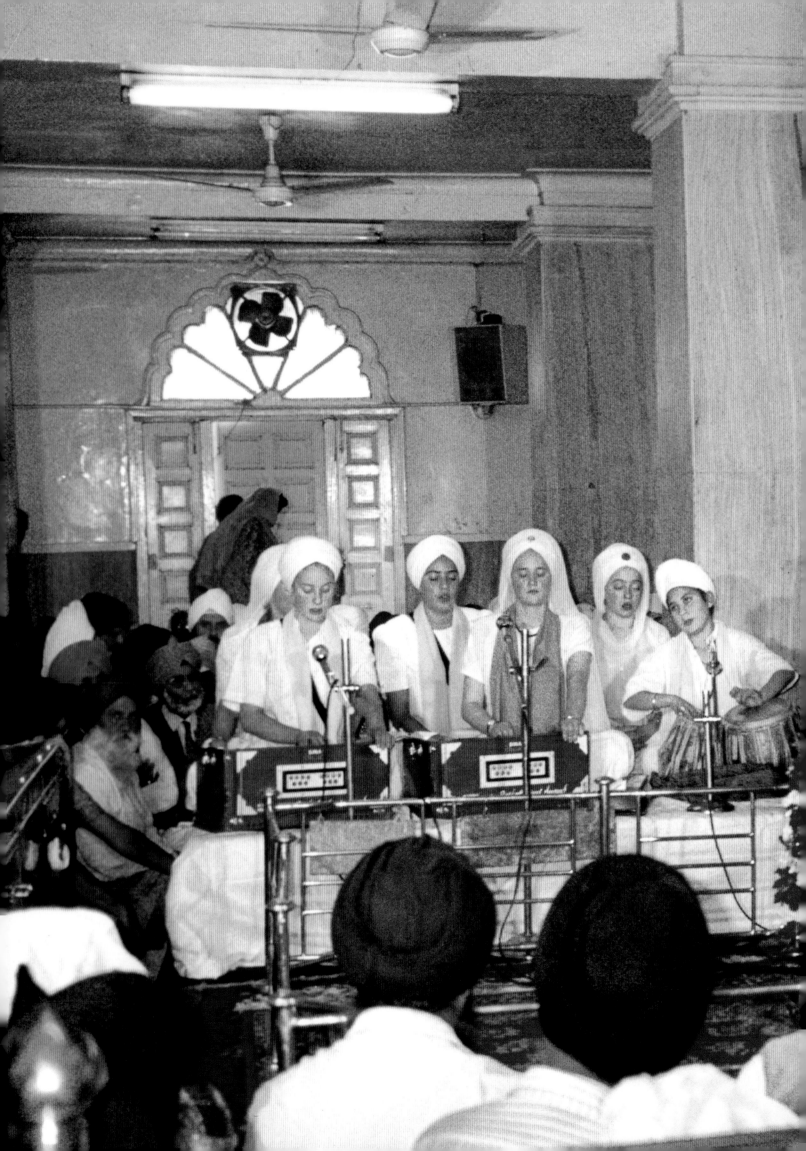

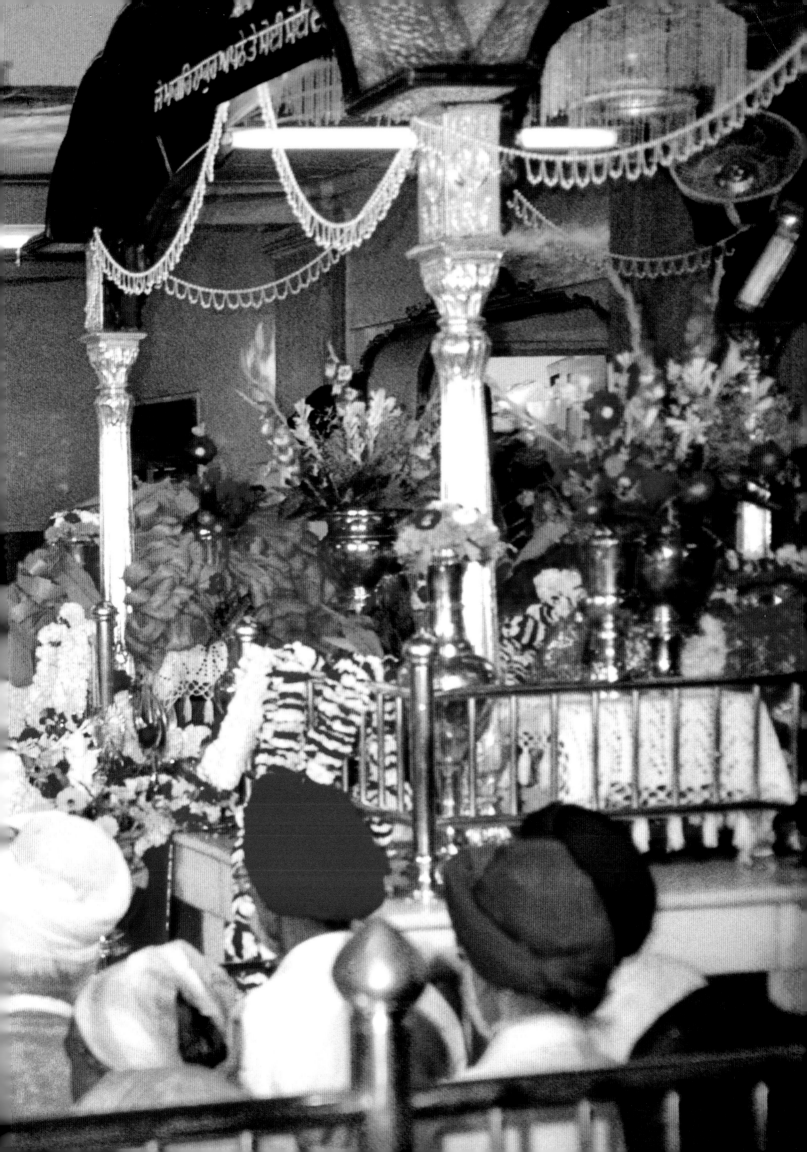

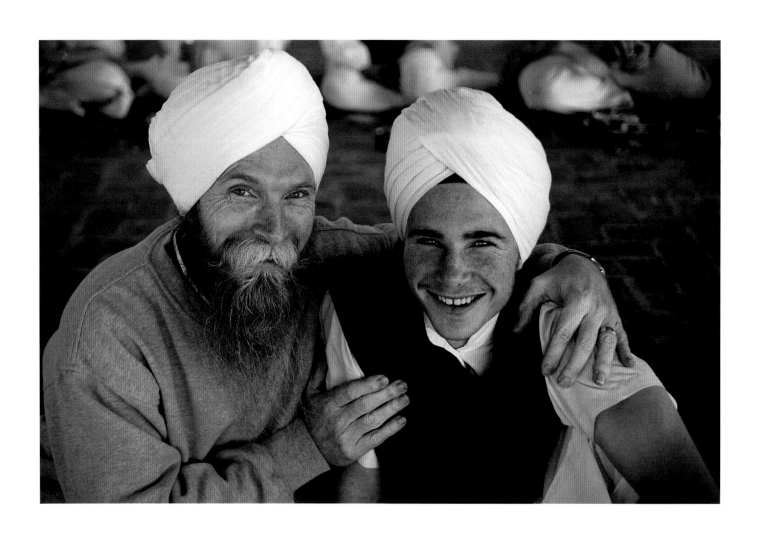

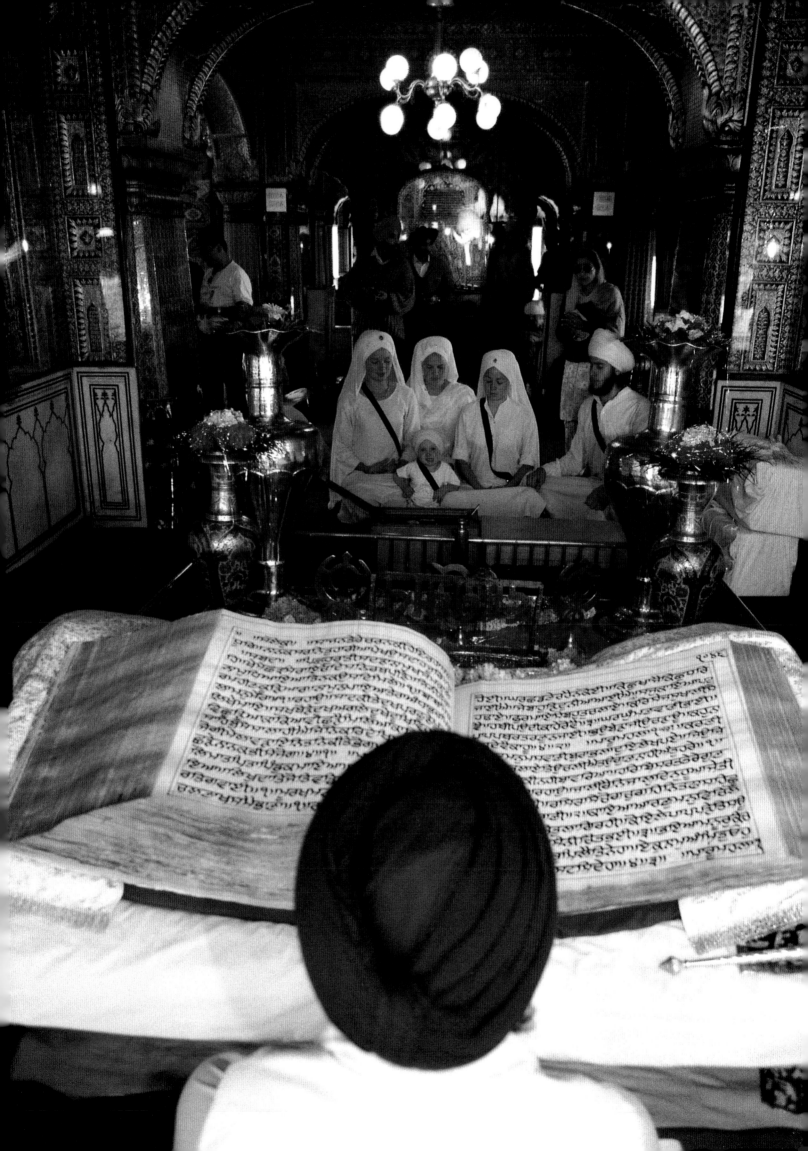

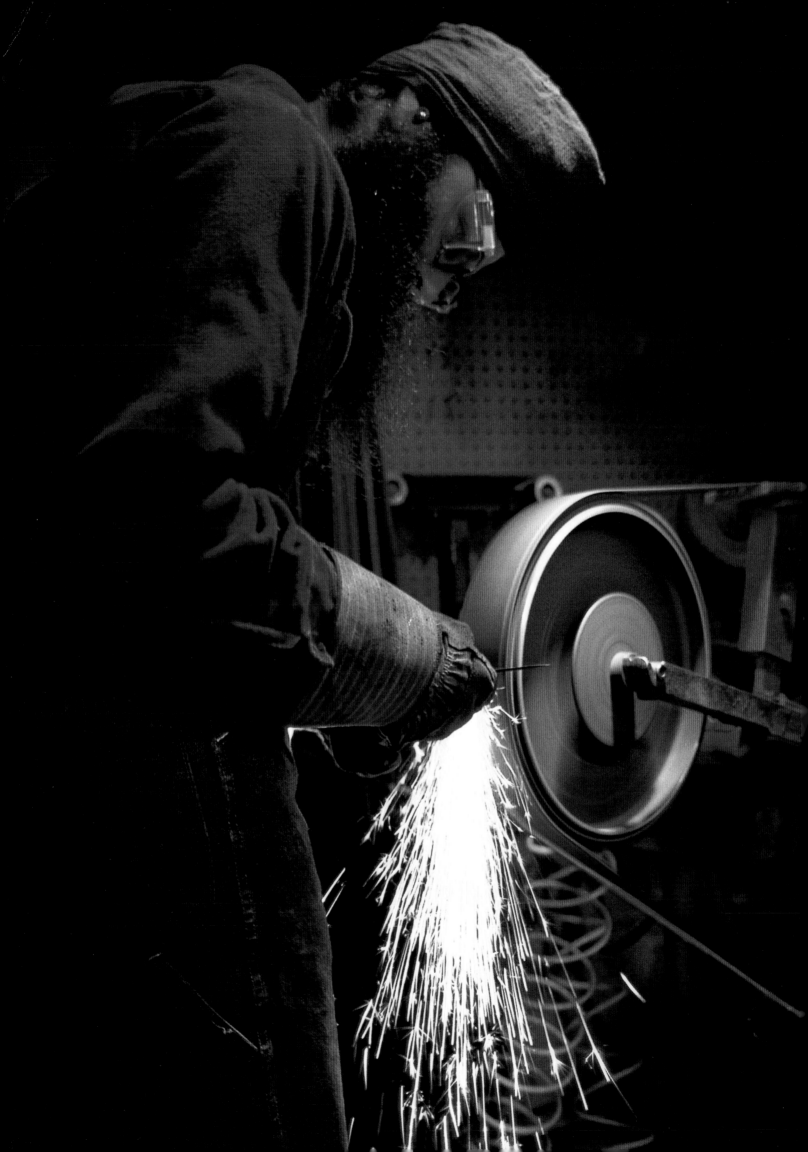

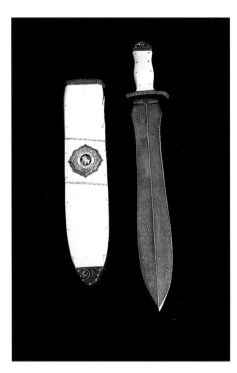

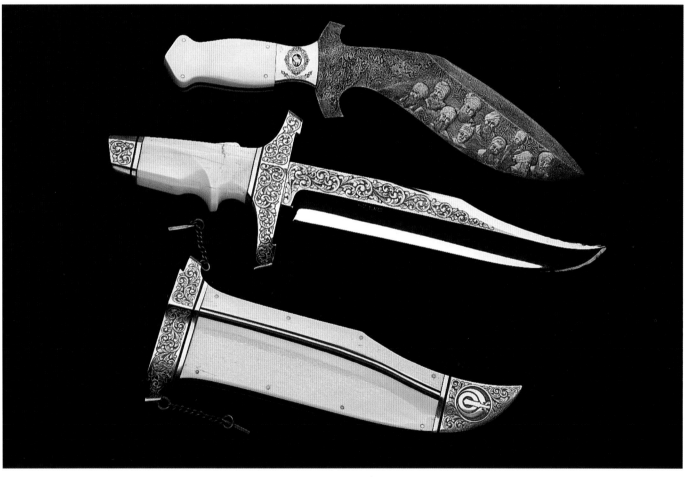

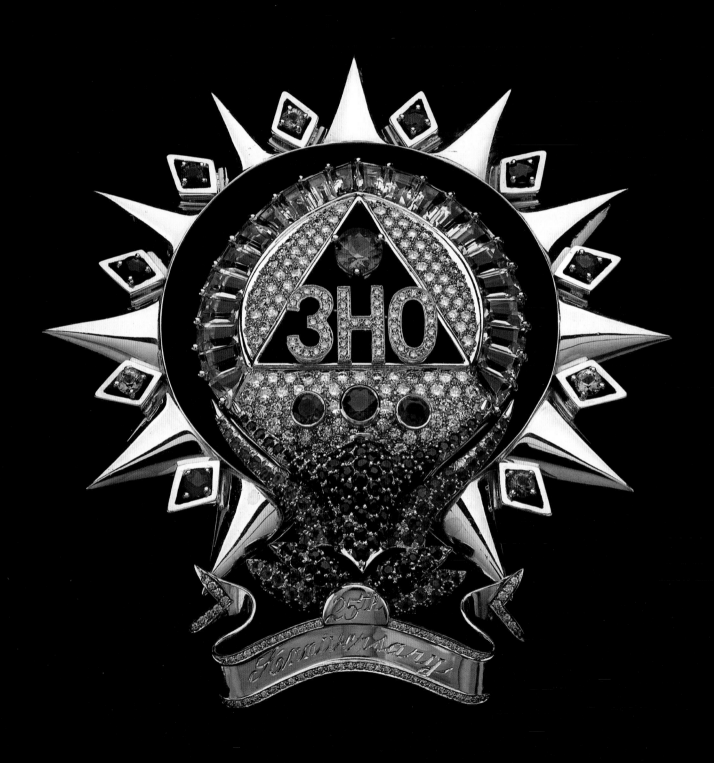

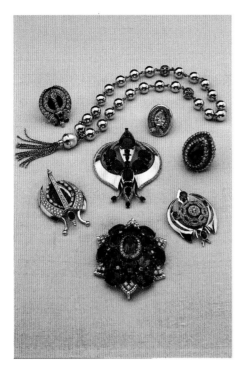

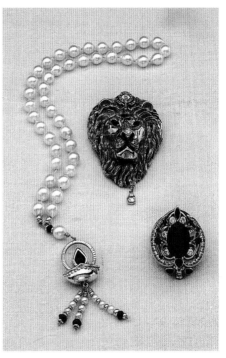

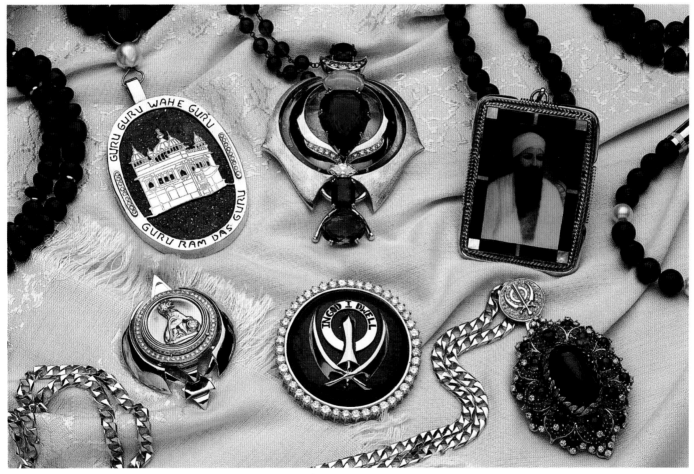

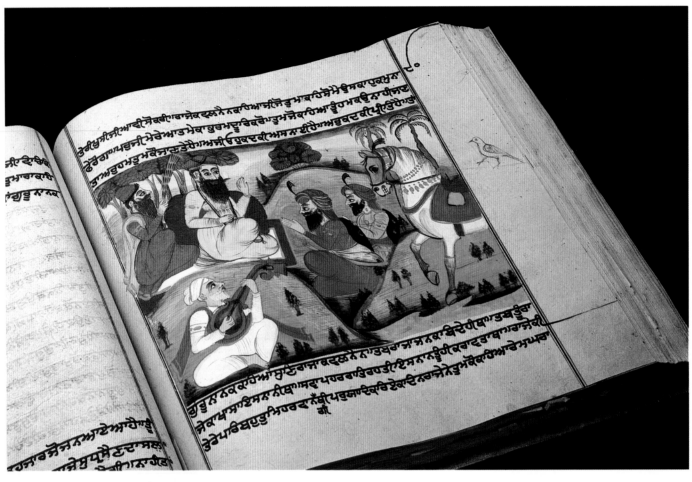

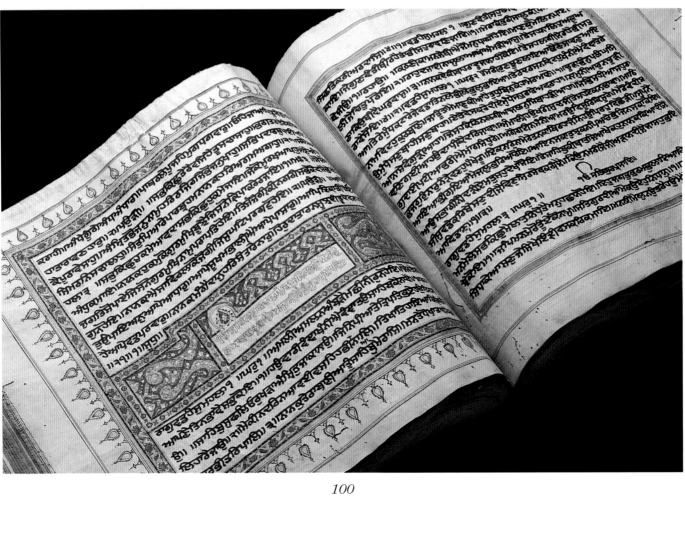

Chapter Three

The Sovereign Khalsa Spiritual Nation 1975-1979

*O**nce a goldsmith came to Guru Gobind Singh and asked him why there need-*
ed to be an established form and discipline, a "Rehit," in the Khalsa of the
Guru. Guru Gobind Singh smiled and told him to come back the following
morning and he would give him the answer.

The next day when the goldsmith returned, Guru Gobind Singh handed him a piece
of gold, and asked him if it was real.

"It looks genuine," replied the goldsmith, "but I need my touchstone to be sure." The
goldsmith brought his touchstone, rubbed the gold, looked at it and said, "There, you see!
This is pure gold."

Guru Gobind Singh asked him, "You have been a goldsmith your whole life. Why
couldn't you tell me right on the spot if this gold was real or not?"

"Sir," he replied, "I am a goldsmith and I know the look, smell, and taste of gold. But
when I want to be one hundred percent sure of its authenticity I use a touchstone."

Guru Gobind Singh said, "To be one hundred percent sure of the authenticity of the
Khalsa, for now and for all times, I also must have a touchstone. My touchstone shall be
the Rehit, which will reveal the purity and perfection of the Khalsa. It is as simple as that."

Chapter Three

Growing from Cubs into Lions

Sikh Dharma of the Western Hemisphere had blossomed with strength and grace into a strong family devoted to the mission of Guru Ram Das. White turbans and long, flowing beards could be seen in nearly every major city in the United States, and the European sangat was growing and prospering. Many of the young Sikhs who began walking the path of Nanak six years ago as wide-eyed teenagers were now husbands and wives responsible for a new generation of children being born to the Khalsa in the West. This collective family proved to be a treasure of talent; art and music were flourishing and businesses were growing.

April 13 is the traditional Baisakhi Day celebration for Sikhs all over the world. But in 1975 in Los Angeles at Guru Ram Das Ashram, a distinct threshold was being crossed. For the first time in history, the Amrit Parchar was being given by a Punj Piare comprised totally of western-born Khalsa. The Punj Piare had prepared themselves with devotion, and were deeply moved by the privilege of serving the sangat in this way. With great reverence they stirred the Amrit water, sweetened with sugar prasad brought all the way from the Golden Temple. As they prepared the Amrit, they were overwhelmed by the depth of the experience and the magnitude of the responsibility they shouldered. That morning they initiated dozens of people into the fold of the Khalsa.

This was a turning point for the growth of the Khalsa in the United States. Prior to this time people saved their money for months, waiting for the opportunity to travel to India to take Amrit at the Akal Takhat. Now the western sangat did not have to wait until they could afford to travel to India before they could be baptized as Khalsa. From this time forward, the Amrit Parchar was held each year at Baisakhi in Los Angeles, Summer Solstice Sadhana in New Mexico, and Winter Solstice Sadhana in Florida. The Siri Singh Sahib was very pleased as he watched the shape and progress of the fulfillment of Guru Gobind Singh's prophecy.

The importance of music continued to grow as part of the 3HO lifestyle, and western Khalsa songs graced every Gurdwara program. These inspiring songs in English touched the hearts of the youth, further ingraining in them the love for the Sikh teachings and their identity as Khalsa. In the spring of 1976, Mukhia Singh Sahib Livtar Singh Khalsa wrote a powerful ballad called the "Song of the Khalsa," which deeply moved the sangat, swelling their hearts with an undefeatable sense of purpose, unity, and destiny. This song encapsulated the strength and spirit of the Khalsa throughout its history and, then as now, it has inspired and uplifted millions of people. At the request of the Siri Singh Sahib, the "Song of the Khalsa" has been sung before the Anand Sahib at all Sikh Dharma Gurdwaras from that time forward.

"One of us put our entire philosophy into one 'Song of the Khalsa.' We shall always sing this with every Ardas and in every congregation to remind ourselves that we must know who we are, what our goal is, and what our concept is. Our will should be like that of steel; our practice should be steady like a mountain; and we should make a mark against the wind of the times to relate that we existed on this planet earth, so that the generations to follow should stand and understand that we excel as a human race."[1]

May 8, 1976 was an unusual Mother's Day in the city of Los Angeles. Organized by Sikh Dharma International Headquarters, a Mother's Day parade, sponsored by the Grace of God Movement, was held to celebrate the spiritual status of women and to protest the exploitation of women in America. About 200 white-clad men, women, and children gathered on the spacious green lawn of the Federal Building in Westwood for the opening ceremonies. Musicians, drummers, an open convertible filled with flowers, and amplified voices singing: "We are the Grace of God," rolled down the streets of Los Angeles. "There we were, smiling and laughing and calling out to the passersby and to the astonished people in the apartment buildings lining our one-mile route, "God Bless you ... Happy Mother's Day ... Sat Nam!"[2]

For the past six years, Sikh Dharma in the West had grown rapidly. Many assets had begun to accrue with hundreds of ashrams and dozens of businesses owned collectively by the people of Sikh Dharma. In order to ensure that this wealth would belong not to any one person but would remain intact for the future generations of the Khalsa, the Siri Singh Sahib of Sikh Dharma Corporation was formed on March 22, 1976 as a nonprofit holding corporation. Properties, vehicles, and the many valuable gifts that were given to Sikh Dharma in the West were enveloped in this corporation.

That summer in Amritsar, the S.G.P.C. discussed the formation, organization, and progress of Sikh Dharma of the Western Hemisphere in their regular committee meetings. The Panthic leadership in Amritsar was enthusiastic and inspired by the resurgence of the Khalsa spirit in foreign countries as the result of the work done by the Siri Singh Sahib. In a vote of support, the Constitution of Sikh Dharma and the Articles of Organization of Sikh Dharma were unanimously endorsed by the Sikh leaders. This endorsement was recorded in their Resolution No. 697 on August 11, 1976. With hospitality and grace, they made plans to receive a large jatha of western Sikhs the following year.

Guru Ram Das Ashrams Grow Roots

The 3HO Ashrams were continuing to grow in strength and numbers, established in nine countries in the Americas, Europe, and Asia. Guru Ram Das Ashrams across Europe prospered and expanded far removed from the 3HO International Headquarters of Los Angeles. The western Sikhs in England, Germany, and Holland succeeded by their own commitment and the strength of their faith and determination. Working across borders, whether they were national, social, spiritual, or prejudicial, they taught yoga classes, fed the hungry, and made a dramatic social impact.

"We have been separated from our spiritual sisters and brothers by thousands of miles, and yet around us here in Europe a family has grown. We are loved in spite of ourselves and our mistakes. Loved for the light which has come through us, even accidentally. Loved for the grace that inherently surrounds those who walk on the Guru's path."[3]

Chapter Three

In London, the people of Guru Ram Das Ashram dedicated their time to serving the local gurdwaras. They served as kirtanis or sevadars working in the langar kitchens. Often they worked with the Sikh youth, inspiring them and encouraging them to maintain the Rehit of Guru Gobind Singh. These young people found a lot in common with each other. The Indian-born sangat received the western Sikhs with warmth and hospitality, and the sangats of London worked together in the Guru's mission.

In Amsterdam, the highly successful Golden Temple Conscious Cookery was well known for its delicious and healthy natural foods. They established a free kitchen that served a hearty meal without charge to the hundreds of young travelers who flocked to the City of Canals in the early seventies. "They say that when we landed in Amsterdam three years ago, people looked at us and laughed in seven languages! If they are still laughing now, it is only because they are feeling the joy and love which has grown in that city under the grace of the House of Guru Ram Das. The day starts in the Amsterdam ashram with wakeup in Punjabi, English, Dutch, French, Spanish, Portuguese, and German. Even then you sometimes have to just shake people awake and point towards the shower! But when the chanting starts, you can see on the faces that they really do understand. If some details were missed, well, it doesn't matter. It'll get worked out."[4]

Hacienda de Guru Ram Das in Española had grown from 11 students to a vibrant sangat of more than 30 families. The ashram had blossomed into 20 acres with several new houses and administrative buildings. A lovely home was purchased, nestled in a grove of tall and shady cottonwood trees on the banks of the Santa Cruz river. It was named the "Gold House" because of its bright yellow stucco, and was used as a dormitory for high school and grade school children who came from all over the country to live in Española and attend McCurdy High School, a nearby private Methodist school. The Siri Singh Sahib's two younger children, Kamaljit Kaur and Kulbir Singh, moved there in 1977 to finish their secondary education. The small town of Española provided them with an opportunity to grow without the overbearing pressures of the public schools in the city.

The original ashram building still served as the center for activities and administration. The dormitory rooms had been transformed into offices, and the single men had moved into the barn. Many of the sangat were now married, and the couples lived in rooms in a building humorously referred to as the "boo-dwara," a building that was later transformed into the langar kitchen. At the request of the Siri Singh Sahib, the sangat at Hacienda de Guru Ram Das held two consecutive Akand Paths in the sadhana room each week. This combined with running the Golden Temple Restaurant and the Golden Temple Healthfood Store in Santa Fe kept the sangat continually busy serving the ashram and integrating into the local business community.

In the humble, white stucco building of Hacienda de Guru Ram Das there was a treasure that surprised and delighted the many visitors. The sadhana room held an ethereal mural depicting the Virgin Mary of Guadalupe surrounded by the ten Sikh Gurus, scenes from their lives, the Golden Temple, and the devout Don Diego on his knees beholding the Lady of Guadalupe. Completed by the celebrated artist Edward O'Brien in 1975, this outstanding work of art is today the east wall of the Takhat-a-Khalsa Gurdwara. He had painted two other murals in New Mexico, one at the St. Katherine's Indian School in Santa Fe, the other at the Pecos Monastery in Pecos, and several more in his home state of Illinois. The love and devotion Mr. O'Brien had for the Virgin Mary transcended the limitations of creed and theology into a pure and universal form.

Mr. O'Brien had been well known to the Sikhs since the early days of the Guru Ram Das Ashram. In his association with the people of the ashram, he had many moving religious discussions and was inspired by their devotional and energetic approach to life. Through the process of his own internal growth and path of self-discovery, he conceived a work of art that combined his love for the Lady of Guadalupe with the lives and fundamental principles of the Sikh Gurus. He started the mural in 1973 in his studio in Santa Fe, and moved to the ashram in 1974 so that he could devote his time to it completely. The mural was finished in the spring of 1975, and he had planned to travel to India in the coming fall to see the Golden Temple and the land of the Sikh Gurus for himself. To the deep sorrow of the Sikhs, who all loved him, Edward O'Brien died at home one week after the mural was finished.

The Siri Singh Sahib said about his work: "This man was able to do what I could never do; he accurately told the history of this world in his painting, and perfectly predicted the events of man up to 5,000 years into the future. O'Brien will be known in the history of man from this time forth and books will be written on his works. Pilgrimages will be made to see his murals and the power of his faith captured in paint."[5]

In the spring of 1975, a rustic ranch was purchased and refurbished as a Sikh Dharma training center and guest housing for Sikh Dharma International staff. Sitting under three beautiful cottonwood trees on over 20 acres of fields, "the Ranch" was soon to be the home of the Siri Singh Sahib whenever he visited Española, which was about four times in 1975. Behind the ranch house, a simple geodesic dome was constructed as a private meditation room for the Siri Singh Sahib. This unique structure was designed and built by the humble hands of Guru Meher Singh of Española. With love and devotion, he worked into the late hours of the night anxiously trying to complete the building before the Siri Singh Sahib came to New Mexico for Summer Solstice. With many other sevadars they created it as a labor of love, donating their time and materials for the construction.

The Khalsa Council Takes the Reins
The Siri Singh Sahib asked that the ministers prepare themselves to carry the responsibility that he now carried; to take up the leadership of Sikh Dharma and give compassion and guidance to the sangat. When the Regional Ministers met on October 24, 1974, he inaugurated them as the "Khalsa Council," and gave them the responsibility as the "Chief Administrative Body of Sikh Dharma in the Western Hemisphere."

In the summer of 1975, the Siri Singh Sahib declared the home of the Khalsa Council to be Hacienda de Guru Ram Das in Española, the "mother ashram" of the 3HO community. Together the members of the Khalsa Council did seva at the Ranch, working with their hands "by the sweat of their brow" to clean up the grounds, prepare the house, and assist Guru Meher Singh in building the Dome.

"Whosoever will do a little seva in this house, God shall stand for that person through every incarnation. If ever I have spoken a truth and you have believed me, you can know that whosoever will serve this house, he shall be served forever. That is why when I find somebody in a tragedy and feeling very miserable, I tell them to go to Hacienda de Guru Ram Das. There is no herb there. There's nothing you can see. I can tell you that Guru Ram Das is everywhere, but he lives in New Mexico. God knows how much shelter the psyche of that place is providing. You have no way to estimate it, but I see how the Unseen showers His grace and blessings on each one there."[6]

That summer the structure and mode of operation of the Khalsa Council were established by the Siri Singh Sahib in a way that was meant to endure, ensuring adherence to the highest letter of the Guru's teachings. "The Khalsa Council is a structure for the present that must stand for the future generations and not be subject to the whims or personality of any one individual but rather be the blueprint for righteous living henceforth."[7]

The basic structure of the Khalsa Council was made up of several sections that acted as an effective system of checks and balances in order to ensure the implementation of righteous decisions. The main body of the Khalsa Council was made of Regional Directors and key administrative personnel from Sikh Dharma International Headquarters Secretariat. The Council of Nominees, separate and distinct from the main body of the Khalsa Council, was a body of 11 sangat members appointed by the Siri Singh Sahib. Their duty was to inspire the Khalsa Council to act with complete fidelity to Sikh Dharma, and to monitor its deliberations for the Siri Singh Sahib. The Council of Nominees could not participate in discussions or vote on issues, but they had the power of veto over any decision of the Khalsa Council and were to report directly to the Siri Singh Sahib their opinions and views. The Bhai Sahib of the Khalsa Council was responsible for interpreting matters of scripture and protocol regarding the religious duties and functions of Sikh Dharma. The Chancellor was responsible for any legal or organizational matters that applied to the Khalsa Council. Working in concert with the Khalsa Council was the "General Sangat," composed of members of the Khalsa Council, Sub-Regional Directors, and individuals selected by the Siri Singh Sahib. The General Sangat met to discuss policy for Sikh Dharma and to provide new ideas and input for the Council.

Tying all these functions together as one unit was the Secretary General, who was responsible for the functioning of the Khalsa Council and the execution of the actions and decision of that body. They met twice a year to discuss and deliberate over the pressing issues of Sikh Dharma.

The Amazing Summer of 1975

Summer Solstice Sadhana in June of 1975 was the beginning of a very busy and exciting period. Time compressed itself that summer, and more was accomplished in those few months than one could think possible. The Summer Solstice Sadhana was held in the mountains of the Pecos Wilderness at an altitude of about 9,000 feet. It was a beautiful, wooded site with two streams running through it and horses and cattle grazing under an endless New Mexico sky. Nearly 1,500 people attended Solstice that year, and there was the usual bustle of activity around the five days of White Tantric Yoga, including ordination of ministers, weddings, and Khalsa Council meetings. On the sixth day of the Solstice camp, 108 people came forward to take the sacred baptism of Amrit and commit their lives to living as Khalsa.

The last three days of the 1975 Solstice were dedicated to the enormous task of hosting the 2nd Annual Unity of Man Conference. Before Sant Kirpal Singh died in September of 1974, he requested that the Siri Singh Sahib carry on the tradition that he had started in India the year before. It was for this request that the Siri Singh Sahib worked with Reno Sirrine, the head of the Ruhani Satsang in the western United States, to make the conference a success in New Mexico. Representatives from every major religion in the world came from India, Mexico, South America, Europe, Japan, and other countries to attend the Unity of Man Conference. Hindus, Jains, American Indians, Jews, Buddhist, Christians, Muslims, and other religions came together in prayer. Workshops were held to discuss solutions to some common problems of achieving practical unity in working for world peace and uplifting human consciousness. The sangat served the guests with the grace and abundance for which Sikhs are universally known.

When the conference was drawing to an end and all the dignitaries were escorted to the airport, the sangat who had worked hard to make it a success longed to breathe a huge sigh of relief. But that was not in the cards. In a spontaneous announcement, the Siri Singh Sahib called all the sangat to remain in Española for a summer course he would teach. Wrapped in a brown shawl and orange turban, the Siri Singh Sahib came out from his Dome to teach daily in the front courtyard of the Ranch under the shade of the tall cottonwood trees. In this eight-week course, later titled "Under the Blue Skies of New Mexico," he revealed many spiritual mysteries including the origin of sound, the power of the Word, and the important role it plays in our lives. He introduced the science of Naad and specified scientific and technical methods of chanting shabads from the *Siri Guru Granth Sahib*. Bhai Sahib Dayal Singh Khalsa also taught Gurmukhi classes, and instructed people in gurdwara protocol and the care of the *Siri Guru Granth Sahib*. In August, Gurucharan Singh Khalsa and the KRI staff taught a Kundalini Yoga teacher's training course on the front lawn of the Ranch. The sleepy ashram of Española had come alive, buzzing with energy and activity.

For the first time, the Siri Singh Sahib celebrated his birthday in New Mexico instead of Los Angeles. More than 1,000 people crowded into the Museum of Fine Arts in Santa Fe to enjoy delicious vegetarian food, birthday cake, and music from the Khalsa String Band. Friends and neighbors from every walk of life came to congratulate the "Yogi" and wish him well.

The Death of a Saint

Bhai Sahib Dayal Singh Khalsa returned to Los Angeles that fall, preparing to travel to India again. He was planning to stay and meditate at the Golden Temple for 40 days, to do seva, and increase his knowledge of Gurbani and the *Siri Guru Granth Sahib*. Together with other devoted young Sikhs, Bhai Sahib was driving from Los Angeles to New York where he was to depart for India and his most beloved Amritsar. With his heart and mind set upon the Golden Temple, he began his journey to the home of his Guru, a journey which would take him not just to the Guru's house, but into the very lap of Guru Ram Das. On September 22, 1975, two months before his 21st birthday, Bhai Sahib Dayal Singh was killed in a car accident. The entire Sikh Panth from all points of the globe was stunned and grief stricken at the loss of Dayal Singh, who was universally loved and respected.

"He was 16 years old when he came to us. He lived totally unto Guru. He was not even 21 when he left his body. His death was not mourned by a handful of friends and known people. His death has become a legend and the entire nation of the Khalsa stood for his prayer. This miracle was accomplished in just five years because he dedicated himself to God and Guru in such a positive way."[8]

His ashes were carried to India in October by a jatha of 50 people. The group was received at the airport by a large delegation of Sikhs who had cooked a beautiful langar and met their western brothers and sisters with a warm welcome. The group then flew directly to Amritsar for the celebration of Guru Ram Das's birthday, and for holy darshan at the Golden Temple.

The jatha later traveled to Kiratpur to disperse the ashes of Bhai Sahib Dayal Singh in the river. His fiancée, Kirn Jot Kaur, carried his ashes and led the procession of barefoot Sikhs who had come to pay him a final tribute along the riverbank. Rowing out onto the river, Kirn Jot lovingly sprinkled his ashes into the water. On the shore, the crowd waited in grief and respect while five shots rang out, echoing through the peaceful countryside in honor of the young American saint.

Most of the group returned to America in December, although a small jatha remained in India to serve the sangat. Called the Guru Ram Das Sikh Seva Jatha, they traveled throughout the Punjab giving kirtan programs and lectures that were received by millions of people. This group participated in the 7th Sikh Youth Camp, sponsored by the Institute of Gurmat Studies. Here they taught yoga and meditation classes, martial arts, and group discussions on the Sikh way of life. After the camp, the jatha taught yoga and meditation classes at the Siri Singh Sahib's home in New Delhi. Nearly 100 Sikh youths joined them each Sunday, and they held meditation classes at the Khalsa Colleges in the area. The jatha returned to the United States in

March of 1976 with a strong vision of their role in India and a desire to carry on the missionary spirit.

These few western Sikhs made a powerful impression on the people of Punjab, and they drew much support and positive attention. However, dark forces were at work in India, and the western Sikhs also drew the attention of people who were not favorable to a full-fledged Sikh renaissance and the implications of greater Sikh strength. In the complicated political profile of the Punjab, the western Khalsa were an unplanned for and disruptive factor in the schemes of those who wished to bifurcate the influence of the Sikhs. Innocently absorbed in their purely missionary efforts, the young Sikhs had no inkling as to this destructive side of Indian politics.

Khalsa Women's Training Camp is Born

Immediately following Summer Solstice Sadhana 1976, the Siri Singh Sahib inaugurated the first Khalsa Women's Training Camp in Española. Women from all over the world were invited to attend this eight-week spiritual camp, set up in the shady cottonwood trees of the Gold House at Hacienda de Guru Ram Das. Mornings were filled with the spirit of martial activities: running the obstacle course, formation marching, martial arts, and rifle shooting. Afternoons were filled with classes and highlighted with a lecture by the Siri Singh Sahib under the gold and white big-top tent.

"Every second of the day in camp was utilized. We ended our sadhana with a mile run. We ate breakfast fast and dashed off to swimming and tennis. We tilled the land in the garden that provided our food. We clambered over the five-foot wall and crawled on our bellies through the dirt of our obstacle course. We learned the noble art of Gatka [traditional Sikh martial art]. At the sound of the bell, we raced to our karate class. Muscles that hadn't even been thought of in years were strengthened."[9]

The Siri Singh Sahib had been a champion for the dignity of the western woman since his arrival seven years earlier. He correctly perceived that the strength of women was critical in the difficult times that lay ahead for the people of the world. "This camp is very important; it will be the basis for you to run future ashrams. You do not have many years left to practice. In a few years you will find tremendous insanity in the streets of this land and you will be in a position to be called upon. You won't be able to do anything through your emotions. Then your sanity, your devotion, your divinity, and your dignity will play the part. Our ultimate aim is to build a purifying woman. A woman should not only be pure, but her presence should cause purification. This process is not going to end, come what may."[10]

News of the exciting 1976 women's camp spread quickly throughout the 3HO family and the summer of 1977 brought more than 200 women to Española. The living conditions were simple and rough, living in tents under the cottonwood trees of the Gold House. But the experience of this beautiful, spiritual sisterhood built an inner strength that many had never before experienced.

The center of the 1978 Khalsa Women's Training Camp was the Siri Singh Sahib's lectures on "The Beaming Faculty of Women." Throughout these lectures, he introduced the women to the concept of nobility as their primary strength and identity. "The greatest decoration a woman can have is nobility. Nobility is a virtue, a living virtue. Some people think if they know manners and pretend to be noble, that they are noble. No, nobility is a character in a woman. A noble woman will give birth to noble environments. A noble woman will give birth to nobility in all areas of life. The sign of nobility is that it has a deep effect in relationship with any person one comes across. They say nobility is a virtue that affects every soul. It is a virtue that affects every soul just as innocence affects every heart. Woman has only one virtue: she is noble in the beginning and noble until her death. If nobility is ever precious to a person, that person will never, ever put herself down for any reason. Because nobility is like a mirror, once a crack is in it the entire image is distorted. Noble habits, noble language, noble behavior, noble posture, and a noble way of communication are so powerfully impressive that even an enemy's heart can be melted."[11]

Nobility became the personification of the Khalsa woman, and the beautiful song "Nobility" was composed from the teachings of the Siri Singh Sahib. It became the theme song of KWTC 1978, and it was being sung by women all over the world.

The Perpetual Traveler

The Siri Singh Sahib's itinerary kept increasing, and he was averaging 200 days of travel annually, teaching more than 45 courses in as many different cities. White Tantric Yoga courses began on Friday evening, continued all day on Saturday, and resumed again on Sunday afternoon, stretching the endurance of the participants and taking a huge toll on the health of the Siri Singh Sahib. Sat Simran Kaur was his travel secretary, scheduling the innumerable appointments, dinners, engagements, and managing the arrangements of his living and transportation. "Always bringing people together in their highest consciousness to recognize the unity of all God's creatures, the Siri Singh Sahib continues on his remarkable travels on this planet. Teaching White Tantric Yoga as only he can do and lecturing in all the gurdwaras along the way, he also meets with the Indian communities to inspire and rekindle in them the fervor and zest for adhering to the basic tenets of Sikh Dharma. A true son of Guru Gobind Singh, he continues to bring hope to the hopeless, courage to the hearts of thousands, and spirit to all people of the earth."[12]

In the spring of 1976 during his Asian tour, the Siri Singh Sahib taught more than 300 Japanese students who participated in courses in Tokyo and Osaka. In Hong Kong, Bangkok, and Singapore, he delivered inspiring lectures about the Sikh Rehit to the sangat, challenging them to take up the discipline of Guru Gobind Singh. After returning to the United States, he left again in May to tour the European Sangats and to teach White Tantric Yoga in Holland and England.

"Wherever he traveled, if there was a gurdwara in that city, he spoke to the sadh sangat, reminding them of the value of the Dharma with which they had been blessed since birth. He urged them not to forsake it, no matter what temptations or pressures they might face. He visited families and urged them to maintain a daily practice of sadhana, paath, and kirtan. He counseled young couples having difficulty in marriage and brought them to reconciliation. He inspired men and women who had lost their faith in their Guru and cut their hair; through his efforts, many returned to the life of Dharma."[13]

Mexico City had a special caliber of students who touched the heart of the Siri Singh Sahib. Whole families came to the White Tantric Yoga courses, aunts and uncles, children, and grandparents. These people had a faith and a humility that brought them many blessings. They called him "maestro," and they felt that just by the touch of his hand on their head, they were healed. Their joy and inspiration brought tears to the eye and warmth to the heart.

The long-awaited Men's Course taught by Yogi Bhajan in 1978 in Boston was an overwhelming success. The urgent requests from the men in the sangat for such a course finally prevailed upon the Siri Singh Sahib, and he started their special training program. This was followed by one in Los Angeles, then a series throughout the next five years. He taught that a man's real strength is not in his physical body, or his personality, but in his capacity to maintain a meditative mind as reflected in a powerful arcline, the outer layer of the auric body. With detailed meditations, foods, and exercises especially for men, he taught men how to heal themselves, creating a blueprint for a strong Khalsa man.

Sikh Dharma Impacts on the World

The year 1977 brought President Jimmy Carter to Washington, DC, and Sikh Dharma was represented in all the religious activities surrounding that event. Interfaith services, ministerial meetings, receptions for clergy, and finally the inaugural ball provided opportunities for people to meet the ministers of Sikh Dharma, to ask questions, and to become familiar with the Sikhs. At the concert called "Minority Perspective," all of the religious communities in America prepared musical and vocal arrangements in praise of God. The musicians of Sikh Dharma presented their beautiful, inspiring music and spoke about the importance of all religious people to work together in spiritual unity.

Through the efforts of the Kundalini Research Institute, the lectures and meditations given by the Siri Singh Sahib were transcribed and printed in manuals and books. By 1977 more than 20 books were in publication. Hawthorn Publications printed two titles of Yogi Bhajan's, making them available for mass distribution: *The Golden Temple Vegetarian Cookbook,* a collection of original recipes used in the Golden Temple Restaurants; and *The Teachings of Yogi Bhajan,* a book of the Siri Singh Sahib's inimitable quotations on the subjects of love, happiness, wisdom, and life. Dr. Sat Kirpal Kaur Khalsa and the sangat in Eugene, Oregon took on the responsibility of transcribing and publishing the lectures from Khalsa Women's Training Camp, and these books made available the Siri Singh Sahib's priceless and unique teachings for and about women.

A new secretariat building was purchased in March of 1977 at 1649 Robertson

Boulevard., to house the growing staff and responsibilities of Sikh Dharma International Headquarters. All the various and makeshift offices were moved out of apartments, living rooms, and garages into this elegant, gracious building that included 11 offices, a lounge, library, and attractive reception area. This was the first Sikh Secretariat ever to be opened anywhere in the world. During the opening ceremonies on August 28, 1977, the Siri Singh Sahib said, "I can assure all of you, our purpose is one thing: to bring peace to all those who seek it and to bring service to all those who need it. I feel proud that the Khalsa as a nation will survive all tests of time and shall live to their tradition and history in service of mankind."[14]

Ram Das Puri is Established in New Mexico

Because the sangat had grown so large, one of the biggest needs was to find a permanent spot that could be developed for the Summer Solstice Sadhana camp. For months different sites were considered, but nothing they had seen fit all the requirements. One day in the spring of 1977 when the Siri Singh Sahib was visiting New Mexico, he was out driving with some people in the sangat when he requested they turn onto a winding dirt road that went into the mountains. After several miles they came onto a flat stretch of road, and he was struck with the beauty and simple, spiritual grace of the high-desert Pajarito Plateau. Standing majestically at an altitude of 7,500 feet, the land had a sweeping panoramic view of the snow-capped mountains and surrounding valleys. When the Siri Singh Sahib looked out over the land, his gaze was held in rapt attention, for he saw a scene that the other people in the car could not behold. In the skies above the plateau he saw a huge gathering of luminous angels, the sight of which made him decide this land was the place for which he had been searching.

Although most of the land in that area was owned by the Indian Pueblos or the Federal Government, they stopped a truck traveling toward them down the dirt road, and asked the driver if there was any private land in the vicinity. As it turned out, the man was a rancher who owned one of the few parcels of private land, situated at the high point of the plateau. After earnest bargaining and negotiations, an agreement was reached on May 13 to purchase the 160 acres of land, as long as water could be found under the arid desert.

However, finding water in this mountainous region was not easy. Geologists were hired to evaluate the land, but they could make no definitive recommendations for drilling. As was the local tradition, a water diviner was brought in to determine where the most fortuitous place to drill might be, but he could not find a place where subsurface water existed. Undaunted by these pessimistic reports, the Siri Singh Sahib selected a place, and the driller set up his rig. After several weeks of drilling, many broken drill bits, and patience that nearly expired, an abundance of clear, clean water was found at a depth of 880 feet. Deep below the aquifer ran a subterranean river of exceptional purity. The purchase was joyously finalized, and the beautiful land was christened "Ram Das Puri."

A flurry of activity began to prepare Ram Das Puri for Summer Solstice Sadhana in June. Huge tanks were installed to provide the camp with adequate water. A generator was set up to provide electricity, and tall mercury vapor lamps were erected for light. Since there was not enough time or money to build a kitchen, only a concrete slab was poured and a walk-in refrigerator was built. The cooks and sevadars prepared the solstice meals in the cool and pure open air. Showers were constructed of wood beams with black plastic stretched over them. An area of land was leveled for meditation, classes, sadhana, and White Tantric Yoga. Straw was spread out on the earth and large white parachutes were erected overhead as shelter from the relentless New Mexico sun. Campers set up their tents at the south end of the property, and walked the half-mile to the meditation area at the north end of the property several times each day. The sun was hot, the rain was torrential, the air was thin, and the water was cold; but everyone was exhilarated to finally have a place they could cherish and develop into a home for the Khalsa.

The European Yoga Festival

In August the Siri Singh Sahib embarked on his European tour, and presided at the European Yoga Festival in the south of France. First established in 1974, this beautiful celebration allowed the growing number of students in Europe the opportunity to attend a solstice-type camp as enjoyed by the sangat in the United States. Crossing all barriers of culture and language, students camped together and participated in yoga classes and the teachings of Sikh Dharma.

In 1978 the highlight of the Festival was the three-day White Tantric Yoga Course taught by the Siri Singh Sahib. Simultaneous translations were given in four languages for his lectures to accommodate the diverse nationalities of the group. Two hundred people from all parts of Europe gathered for ten days in the beautiful site of the Chateau La Cloutiere near the town of Loches in France. The festival's program included workshops in meditation and music, kinesiology, massage, martial arts, Gurbani Kirtan, and Gurmukhi.

The beauty and uniqueness of this Yoga Festival was in its international atmosphere. People from different countries and cultures, speaking different languages, came together to share the inspiring path of higher consciousness. Seeing people come from as far north as Scandinavia and as far south as Rome, overcoming the barriers of frontiers, language, and culture was a sign of the commitment of the students in Europe to live to the ideal of a Healthy-Happy-Holy way of life.

Yoga and Sikh Dharma

The practice of Kundalini Yoga in Sikh Dharma was astonishing for many Indian-born Sikhs. In general, Sikhs in India had not retained the practice of yoga as part of their religious identity, and therefore they questioned its place in Sikh Dharma. However, the western Khalsa viewed it as a logical and well-documented part of the Sikh technology, as many of the Sikh Gurus could be seen as masters of yoga. Numerous technical references are found in the *Siri Guru Granth Sahib* using yogic terms to describe the inner life of a Sikh. As described by Guru Gobind Singh, yoga is a key to unlocking the mysteries of God.

Rey man eh bidh jog kamaa-o.

Singhee saach akapat kanthalaa dhiaan bibhoot charaa-o.

Taattee gao aatam bas kar kee, bhichha naam adhaarang.

Baajay param taar tat har ko, upajai raag rasaarang.

Ughatai taan tarang rang at giaan geet bandhaanang.

Chak chak rehe dev daanav mun chhak chhak bayom bivaanang.

Aatam upades bhes sanjam ko, jaap so ajapaa jaapai.

Sadaa rehai kanchan see kaayaa, kaal na kabahoo beyaapai.

O my mind, practice Yoga in this way:

Let Truth be your horn, sincerity your necklace,

and meditation the ashes you apply to your body.

Make self-restraint your harp, and the Name of God your support.

Vibrate the strings of the Sound-Current, and listen to the sweet

songs of the Lord. The waves of sweet sound bring ecstasy,

and through the Songs of the Lord, spiritual wisdom arises.

The demons and the demi-gods in their chariots are amazed,

and the silent sages are intoxicated with delight.

So instruct your soul; wear the loin-cloth of self-restraint,

and chant the Name of the Lord, even when you are silent.

In this way, your body shall remain forever golden,

and death shall never even approach you.

Guru Gobind Singh Ji, Dasam Granth

In this shabad, the essence of the Sikh experience is taught through yogic technology and methodology.

Kundalini is the term used for the potential spiritual energy that resides in every human being. The process of "awakening the kundalini" is the natural process of spiritual growth within the individual. It is referred to by many different names in different religious traditions, but the essence of any experience of the soul is what is referred to as the "rising of the kundalini."

Kundalanee surjhee sat sangat parmaanand Guru mukh machaa.

Siree Guru saahib sabh oopar man bach karam seveeai sachaa.

Through the Word of the Guru, the Kundalini rises in the Sat Sangat and they enjoy the Lord of Supreme Bliss.
The Great Guru is the Lord of all, so serve the True Guru in thought, word and deed.

Siri Guru Granth Sahib Ji, pg. 1402

This rising of the kundalini was referred to in the days of Guru Gobind Singh as "Cherdi Kala." When spiritual energy is high, drenching the Sikh with love of God and Guru, this is the state of Cherdi Kala. As described by the Siri Singh Sahib: "When you do Kundalini Yoga, it is a simple, direct experience, and the kundalini rises. It affects you in spite of all your garbage, so that you start looking toward infinity. That is Cherdi Kala. 'I am I am. Nothing can budge me. Nothing. I am not going to give in. I am all right.'"

Guru Ram Das was known as the master of Raj Yoga. The western Sikhs unreservedly embraced yoga in the style and teachings of Guru Ram Das.

Sabh bidh maaniyo man tab hee bheyo prasan,
Raaj yog takhat dian Gur Raam Daas

When His Mind was totally satisfied in every way, and when He was totally pleased, the throne of Raj Yog was bestowed upon Guru Ram Das.

Siri Guru Granth Sahib, pg. 1399

The Raj Yoga of the Sikh Gurus was different from the traditional practices of yoga in India in three main ways. Guru Nanak counseled the Nath Yogis in the Sidh Gosht, objecting to their practice of renunciation and celibacy. He explained that "Grisht Ashram," or the life of the householder, is the highest destiny and the natural course for a human being. One must earn one's living righteously and share it with others, facing the problems of life as they arise instead of running away from them. To renounce domestic life is to shirk the responsibility of human existence. Guru Nanak criticized the escape from life into the mountains of the Himalayas as a rejection of social responsibilities. He explained that renunciation is an attitude of the mind, not a condition of a particular location or altitude. For without experiencing human love and family responsibilities, it is difficult to realize divine love. He explained this as "Sahaj Yoga," the yoga of the natural existence of human life.

Guru Nanak went on tell the yogis to refrain from trying to reach God through bodily austerities, tortures, and mortifications. He said that this human form was a gift from God and a vehicle of enlightenment, not an enemy to be beaten and subdued. He taught that by chanting God's Name the real yoga can be obtained, and effortlessly so.

The Sikh Gurus also evolved the yogic principle of "Ahimsa," or nonviolence, into a new dimension of the "Sant Sipahi," the soldier-saint. Since the time of the sixth Guru, Guru Hargobind, the Sikhs had taken up the sword for the righteous defense of the weak and oppressed. The teachings of Guru Gobind Singh to his Khalsa are very specific in the use of arms, and he stated that "Only after all peaceful means have failed is it legitimate to take up the sword in defense of righteousness."

Bhai Gurdas, an eminent Sikh writer, describes the Sikh as a perfect yogi, a goal which the western Sikhs hold high:

> *The Sikh is a living yogi, unattached in the midst of maya.*
> *The Guru's mantra is his earrings, the dust of saintly feet is his holy*
>   *ashes.*
> *His cloak is practical humility; the Sat Sangat is his spiritual*
>   *sustenance.*
> *He blows the horn of the Guru's shabad; his staff is divine*
>   *knowledge.*
>
> Bhai Gurdas[15]

The Strength and Grace of Sikh Dharma

As a service to the community, Kundalini Yoga teachers across the United States started offering yoga classes in prisons. In the prison world, where there is little love or positive communication and a constant struggle for emotional and physical survival, the science of yoga and meditation was a rare opportunity for peace and relaxation. By 1979 there were well over 100 yoga programs in local, state, and federal correctional institutions throughout the country. Many of the staff and inmates who attended the classes said that through Kundalini Yoga and contact with the Sikhs, they found a new peace of mind and joy in living.

In his continuing efforts to promote unity in the various religious communities, on August 7, 1977, the Siri Singh Sahib participated in the Spiritual Life Jubilee, a celebration of religious unity sponsored by Wallace D. Muhammed, chief Imam of the World Community of Al-Islam. For the first time in the history of the Sikhs, the sangat worked alongside their Muslim brothers and sisters staging an event in praise of the One God. It was a surprise and a pleasure for the sangat to see all the graceful Muslim ladies in their beautiful white turbans!

On October 25, 1979, the Dalai Lama came to meet the Siri Singh Sahib at the Guru Ram Das Ashram in Los Angeles. This was the first of many visits and an instant rapport sprung up between these two religious leaders. The Dalai Lama as the spiritual head of Tibetan Buddhism, was forced into exile in 1959 by Communist China. Under Communist suppression, temples were closed, religious artifacts and scriptures were destroyed, and monks were slaughtered. The Dalai Lama and his people took refuge in India, and the Sikhs played a host role in his exodus.

The Siri Singh Sahib spoke of the friendship between the Sikhs and the Tibetan

Buddhists. He expressed his gratitude to the Tibetan Buddhists for the role they have played over hundreds of years in maintaining a spiritual equilibrium in the magnetic-field of the earth. He spoke warmly about the historical documents kept by the Tibetans, recording the history of the world for thousands of years. The Siri Singh Sahib and the Dalai Lama would meet several times in the coming years, always exhibiting the strength of their friendship and their common mission in the service of mankind.

In order to support the expanding responsibilities of Sikh Dharma International Headquarters, the financial requirements were tremendous. In the historical tradition of the Sikhs, the system of Das Vand was instituted in September of 1978 to meet these expanding needs. Each member of Sikh Dharma was requested to contribute 10 percent of his or her earnings for the growth of the mission. These monies were budgeted to support the Regional Centers, Khalsa schools and youth programs, missionary programs, free kitchens, publications, and the Secretariat of Sikh Dharma. "All of my life I have believed in one thing: anything you give in the Name of God returns to you ten times. That is my personal experience. That is why I can tell you and I can share with you: I believe in giving; I live by giving."[16]

In honor of the ten-year anniversary of 3HO Foundation and 50th birthday of the Siri Singh Sahib, a gala banquet was held on September 1, 1979, at the Beverly Wilshire Hotel in Los Angeles with over 600 people in attendance. The event, "Ten Years of Serving People," was a once-in-a-lifetime celebration. The Siri Singh Sahib was honored by his students and friends for a decade of work and devotion to the mission of Guru Ram Das in the West. A beautiful book, *The Man Called the Siri Singh Sahib*, was presented to him chronicling the amazing and divine progress of the first ten years of 3HO. There were singing, poetry, and comical skits. The love of thousands of people was displayed as a tribute to the strength and unity of the western sangat.

The Siri Singh Sahib addressed the sangat with deep emotion and gratitude for the efforts of so many Gursikhs. He said, "Ten years after those first few people began to practice this yoga, ten years after the first few students began following this discipline, now we comprise a race of people who walk tall and stand proud. We no longer talk of planting the seeds of a spiritual nation, now we speak of setting the roots. This tenth anniversary represents a coming of age. It gave a concise picture of everything we've been. But more than that, it shows the image of who we are now, and what we are to become."

The Yatra to India in 1977

In the fall of 1977, over 100 people participated in the yatra to India to celebrate the 400th anniversary of the founding of Amritsar. Staying in the Golden Temple guest house, Guru Nanak Nivas, western Sikhs became a familiar sight around the vicinity of the Harimandir Sahib. In the Amrit Vela before the start of the Asa di Var, the group would gather on the roof of the Golden Temple. Sitting together, they chanted *Guru Guru Wahe Guru Guru Ram Das Guru* with love and joy, celebrating the experience of ecstasy of Guru Ram Das. Then they would fill the Golden Temple with bright faces in white bana, listening to the beautiful notes of the Asa di Var. After the coming of dawn, they returned to Guru Nanak Nivas where they had a Kundalini Yoga class on the roof with the splendor of the Golden Temple within sight on the horizon.

As a special prayer for unity and protection of the Sikhs, in the morning and evening the group would walk in double file around the parkarma chanting the Mul Mantra. Many people looked on with surprise and awe, but other Sikhs joined the group in friendship and brotherhood on their march around the parkarma.

With four full buses, the western jatha toured the historical gurdwaras in Punjab offering kirtan programs and speeches. Everywhere they went they were met with an outpouring of love and appreciation, served Guru's langar, and enjoyed the company of the sadh sangat. This huge company of white-dressed Sikhs was living testimony to the impact of the Guru's work in the West.

Traveling into the mountains of the Himalayas, the western jatha made the yatra to Sri Hemkunt Sahib. High in the mountains at this place known as Sipat Saring, Guru Gobind Singh meditated before his birth. The steep ascent, especially the last stretch of stone steps, pushed the endurance of all the yatris. The conquering of fatigue and extreme altitude, finalized by bathing in the icy cold waters of the lake at Sri Hemkunt Sahib reaped great rewards of inner spiritual revelation. The jatha sat in meditation in the mountain gurdwara with a deep love of Guru Gobind Singh.

Many of the western Sikhs made close friendships with the Bhai Randhir Singh jatha. The western Sikh women had never encountered other Sikh women who wore turbans, and this special attribute they had in common stimulated conversations that developed into friendships. Deeply committed to kirtan, mediation, and love of Guru, the western Sikhs found a great sense of kinship with them.

Bhai Fauja Singh, a prominent figure in the Bhai Randhir Singh jatha, was in prison at that time. He had been jailed over a pending case, but moreover was being kept in prison as a means of containing his powerful leadership of the Sikhs. Already in Punjab, a storm of death and tragedy was brewing that would soon engulf all those who called themselves Sikhs of the Guru. Nonetheless, his spirits always remained high and his wife Amarjit Kaur often visited the western jatha at Guru Nanak Nivas with words of support, appreciation, and encouragement. Arrangements were made and many of the western jatha went to the jail to play Gurbani Kirtan for the prisoners there, and to have a chance to visit with Bhai Fauja Singh.

During this time, the Siri Singh Sahib was on a missionary tour of the countries of the far east, visiting the Sikhs in Thailand, Malaysia, Hong Kong, and Japan. He traveled on to Iran and Afghanistan, delivering a message of hope and strength to the devoted sevadars who maintained the historical gurdwaras in those countries and raised their families as Sikhs against difficult odds. On October 27, 1977, the Siri Singh

Sahib flew in from Kabul to join the jatha in Amritsar. He was met at the airport by the Sikh leadership and given a glorious reception. Over one million people had come to Amritsar to celebrate the anniversary of that city; it was unbelievably crowded. The Siri Singh Sahib made his way to the Golden Temple to humbly bow his head and spend a few precious hours there.

From Amritsar, the Siri Singh Sahib traveled up to the Pakistani border, and crossed once again into the Punjab of his birth. Exactly 30 years to the day the Siri Singh Sahib led his village across the Pakistani border into India during the time of partition, he crossed back again, bringing with him a small group of western Sikhs. The Siri Singh Sahib and the jatha visited Nankana Sahib Gurdwara. Here he offered prayers for the return of this historical gurdwara into the hands of Gursikhs, and for the freedom for Sikhs from India to visit this birthplace of Guru Nanak.

On the evening of Guru Ram Das's birthday, they drove through the streets of Lahore to a small building where the Guru was born. Through a large wooden door and up a flight of cement stairs they went into a room where the mother of Guru Ram Das had given birth to a son, Jetha, 440 years before. In the filtered moonlight they said a prayer of gratitude for the blessing this earth had received by the birth of Guru Ram Das. A dream had been fulfilled for the Siri Singh Sahib, who had prayed that God should bless him one day to be at this site on the birthday of his Guru.

As the busy year of 1977 came to a close, the Siri Singh Sahib spoke to the sangat in a lecture: "I am waiting for the day when my dear cubs will roar and let the world know they are committed out of their hearts. It will be far superior that they will get a time to prove their excellence. Steel is always known in the battle, and man is always known against the odds." Unknown to the politically innocent hearts of the western Khalsa, the time to test that steel was rapidly approaching.

The 1978 Martyrs of Amritsar

The jatha returned to America strengthened and uplifted by the experience in India. The bond of friendship between the Bhai Randhir Singh jatha and the western Sikhs served to lighten hearts on both sides of the ocean. In letters to their new brothers and sisters, Bhai Fauja Singh and Amarjit Kaur gave words of encouragement for the work of the Sikhs in the West.

With a prophetic sense of the future, Bhai Fauja Singh wrote in a letter in 1977: "Firstly, with the grace of Guru, one gets knowledge of His Nam in the good company of the Khalsa. He doesn't mind opposition if they oppose him. He does not mind death for the true cause. It is profitable, enjoyable, and pleasurable to him to cost him his life for this end. This is really healthy, happy and holy for him!"

On Baisakhi, 1978, Bhai Fauja Singh led a group of Sikhs to peacefully protest against the Nirankaris who were slandering the Sikh Gurus and insulting the *Siri Guru Granth Sahib.* Though they went with no aggression, each one of them also went knowing that it is the Guru's blessing to give one's life in defense of the honor, dignity, and purity of the *Siri Guru Granth Sahib.* These 100 peaceful protesters were ambushed with a deadly barrage of machine gun fire, acid soaked bricks, and other brutal weapons. Thirteen Khalsa Sikhs were massacred in this way, and up to 80 others were grievously injured. Bhai Fauja Singh lay among the dead.

When the news of the tragedy first reached the United States, the Khalsa Council was in session. The body of the Khalsa Council, most of whom knew Bhai Fauja Singh personally, was stunned as the bloody details were exposed. The meetings were immediately halted and Ardas was offered for those who had given their lives on the streets of Amritsar. The Executive Committee elected to send three representatives to India to honor the martyrs, console the injured, and report on the situation firsthand. Across the United States, the shock and brutality of this event rocked the Sikh communities. Through lectures, letters, and publications, the western Khalsa protested this barbarous, needless violence.

Sikh Dharma and Mother India

The annual yatra to India and Sri Hemkunt Sahib was now a regular event for 3HO in the fall. The white bana and turbans of the western Sikhs became commonplace in the bazaars of Amritsar and in the Amrit Vela at the Harimandir Sahib. In the fall of 1978 and again in 1979, a western jatha returned to India. In a letter written by Sada Sat Kaur Khalsa, she describes with love her experience at the Golden Temple: "One of my favorite times is to be at the gate just before it opens in the morning. When the gong is rung, I feel like that sound is calling all the souls on earth and in the heavens to come in to sit in the sadh sangat in this holy place. My feet, which I am so blessed to have, can hardly carry me fast enough over the threshold and down the walkway to the House of Guru Ram Das Ji. How blessed are those birds that live on the roof and the fish that live in the nectar tank; they are always in that vibration!"

In September of 1979, Vikram Singh Khalsa, Ajeet Singh Khalsa, and Guru Sangat Singh Khalsa were the first Americans to have the privilege of playing kirtan in the Golden Temple. The whole western jatha was there to sing with them, pouring from their hearts the beautiful shabads of the Guru. They played on Guru Ram Das's birthday, which held a special meaning for them.

The western Sikhs traveled extensively throughout the rustic villages of Punjab. They were inspired by the simple devotion and uncompromising ideals of the Punjabi people, and they in turn inspired the Sikh villagers with a vision of the Khalsa beyond the borders of India. Some of the Americans were able to give lectures in the Punjabi language, crossing the linguistic gap that separated east from west.

In the village of Harianwelam, Baba Nihal Singh had heard stories of these western-born Khalsa. Baba Nihal Singh was a brave Jathadar of the Tarana Dal, a jatha of Nihung Sikhs who are traditional soldier-saints of the Khalsa. He was told the western Khalsa held a deep love of Guru and that they were preaching a revival of the Rehit of Guru Gobind Singh. He decided he would meet them, and so with a group of his

Nihungs he traveled to Anandpur Sahib. He and his Sikhs camped at the gates of Anandpur Sahib for more than a week waiting, sometimes impatiently, for the westerners to come. When the jatha did finally arrive, he invited them all to his village. The jatha had a very busy schedule, however, and the group organizers tried to deflect the invitation. Few people are strong enough to say "no" to the Nihungs of Baba Nihal Singh, and to the delight of the jatha he took them all to Harianwelam, showing them the hospitality of a Gursikh village.

The bus drove them deep into the forest and it was dark when the jatha arrived, but the village was ablaze with torches and lanterns to welcome them. Each person was honored with saropas tied on their turbans and gifts of kirpans, Nitnems, and malas. They spent the night playing kirtan and rejoicing in the exalted spirit that a Gursikh derives from the company of the sadh sangat. As if they had been transported through time to the days of Guru Gobind Singh, the western Sikhs were immersed in the customs and discipline of the Nihungs. It was an experience that opened the doors of their souls.

In a subsequent visit, Baba Nihal Singh presented Dr. Sat Kirpal Kaur Khalsa with a *Dasam Granth* that she received on behalf of Sikh Dharma of the Western Hemisphere. This was the first *Dasam Granth* to be given to the Sikhs in the West, and it was an event of great excitement.

Throughout the yatra, the western jatha was constantly confronted with the quickly changing political scenario in India. The Baisakhi massacre in Amritsar was followed in 1978 by more deaths in Kanpur and New Delhi at the hands of the Nirankaris. The question on the lips of every concerned Sikh was: What can we do to stop this?

"We cannot allow the disunity of a few or the slander of the many to hinder the growth of the light of Truth. Nor can we allow the great sacrifices of the martyred Khalsa brothers and sisters go in vain. Now is the time to call on God and Guru to bless us with the strength to live in perfect commitment to the Rehit Maryada, to rise daily in Amrit Vela and repeat the Nam, to experience the nobility and grace of bana, to hold God in our hearts at every moment of the day. It is only by the Grace of God that we will stand strong as steel, steady as stone, to serve and inspire to righteousness all seekers and protectors of Truth."[17]

The Sovereign Khalsa Spiritual Nation

As the decade came to a close, Sikh Dharma had fully taken its place in the world community of the Sikhs. Known throughout the world for the strength of their values, and for upholding the mission of the Gurus against all odds, the western Khalsa had established itself and its place in history. Throughout 1979, the political climate of India moved closer to the brink of what was to be the bloody tragedy of 1984. The atmosphere in the holy city of Amritsar was rapidly changing. Political bickering, continuous treachery, and underlying fear had become a reality of life within the Sikh leadership in India. For this reason, Sikh Dharma took a bold step declaring itself sovereign: free and independent from the dictates and political agendas of others. With their own organizational network and their own governing body of the Khalsa Council, they bowed their heads only to the Creator, and proclaimed themselves free and independent of the boundaries of man. In this declaration, they emerged as the Sovereign Khalsa Spiritual Nation.

As a special representative from the S.G.P.C. in Amritsar, Bhai Sahib Kapur Singh attended the April, 1979 session of the Khalsa Council to assess the Sikhs of the West and bring a report back to Amritsar. An eminent and highly respected Sikh historian and scholar, he attended the meetings, living, eating, and praying with the people of Sikh Dharma. What he saw warmed his heart, and he found hope for the future in the straightforward and dedicated Khalsa of the West. He addressed the assemblage to express his appreciation for the work done by the Siri Singh Sahib in the missionary task God had given him. Cognizant of the hazy motivation and growing duplicity in Amritsar, he wholeheartedly endorsed their declaration of sovereignty.

"Never in the history of Sikhism has it been demanded, or has it been accepted by the body of the Khalsa, that they should be put under police regimentation or that some central authority in control of certain individuals should dictate to them as to how they are to behave. The only allegiance of a true Khalsa and of a true Sikh is to the doctrine and to God, to the Guru and to Truth. Guru Gobind Singh, when he left this world said, 'Henceforth the authority of the doctrine and the destiny rest with Guru Granth, and the determination of policy is with the body of the Khalsa'—not with any centralized regimented body, but the body of the Khalsa. What is Khalsa? Guru Gobind Singh said, 'Wherever five Sikhs who are fully committed to the doctrines of the Guru and who live according to the teachings of the Gurus, in their meditation concentrate on the Guru, that is the Khalsa.'" [18]

The Khalsa Pledge

I pledge allegiance to the Sovereign Khalsa Spiritual Nation, which shall live to obey the Will of God, serve humanity with love and peace, and spread the radiance of the Holy Nam as given by Guru Nanak, through Guru Gobind Singh, and embodied in the Siri Guru Granth Sahib. So that the children of the Khalsa, and all their generations to follow may ever live in the spiritual sovereignty of Khalsa.

The Siri Singh Sahib then stood to address the Khalsa Council: "Holy congregation of the Sat Guru, *Siri Guru Granth Sahib,* this is a day of liberty, and a day of leaving the field of treachery and betrayal to declare ourselves an independent spiritual nation of the Khalsa. We shall be what Guru Gobind Singh in his words said for us to be. Beyond national boundaries is the concept of the Khalsa. We have no political allegiance because we have no seat to win. Our mission is simply to serve humanity and to conquer the heart of every human being so that this world can live Healthy, Happy, and Holy. As our extended goal does not recognize boundaries and restrictions, so we do not recognize boundaries. We are free."[19]

Notes

1. Yogi Bhajan; Feb. 13, 1977, Columbus, Ohio
2. Shakti Parwha Kaur Khalsa; *Beads of Truth*, 1976
3. Gurudain Singh; *Beads of Truth*, 1975
4. Gurudain Singh; *Beads of Truth*, 1975
5. Yogi Bhajan; *Beads of Truth*, Fall 1975
6. Yogi Bhajan; *Beads of Truth*, Fall 1975
7. Yogi Bhajan; *Beads of Truth*, Fall 1975
8. Yogi Bhajan; *Beads of Truth*, 1976
9. Hari Har Kaur Khalsa; *Beads of Truth*, 1976
10. Yogi Bhajan; *Beads of Truth*, 1976
11. Yogi Bhajan; Khalsa Women's Training Camp lecture, July 3, 1978
12. *Beads of Truth*; Summer 1976
13. Shakti Parwha Kaur Khalsa; *The Man Called the Siri Singh Sahib,* pg. 122
14. *Beads of Truth*, Fall 1977
15. Bhai Gurdas, Var 29, 15; *Guru Ram Das; His Life, Work and Philosophy* by Dr. Gobind Singh Mansukhani
16. Yogi Bhajan
17. Nirinjan Kaur Khalsa; *Beads of Truth* Winter 1978
18. Bhai Sahib Kapoor Singh; Khalsa Council, April 1979
19. Yogi Bhajan; Khalsa Council, 4/22/79

SONG OF THE KHALSA

by Mukhia Singh Sahib Livtar Singh Khalsa

1) Many speak of courage, speaking cannot give it,
It's in the face of death we must live it.
When things are down and darkest,
That's when we'll stand tallest.
Until the last star falls,
We won't give an inch at all!

Stand as the Khalsa, strong as steel, steady as stone;
Give our lives to God and Guru, mind and soul, breath and bone.

2) Guru Arjun gave his life to stand for what was right.
He was burned and tortured five long days and nights.
He could have stopped it anytime just by giving in.
His strength a solid wall; he never gave an inch at all!

Sons of the Khalsa, remember those who died;
Stood their ground until their last breath so we who live now might live free lives.

3) A princess is not royal by her birth or blood inside,
But if her family's home is Anandpur Sahib,
She'll walk with such a grace and strength the world will bow in awe.
Until the mountains fall, she won't give an inch at all!

Daughters of the Khalsa, in your strength our future lies,
Give our children fearless minds to see the world through the Guru's eyes.

4) On Baisakhi day we were thousands, but only five had the courage for dying;
One brave man, one flashing sword, turned us all to lions.
And now we live his legacy, to die before we fall;
And like the five who answered his call, we can't turn back at all!

Stand as the Khalsa, strong as steel, steady as stone;
Give our lives to God and Guru, mind and soul, breath and bone.

4) The tenth Guru gave even his sons to give the Khalsa life.
His words stand like mountains against the winds of time;
That Khalsa will rule the world; all will be safe in its fold.
But if the Khalsa falls, there won't be a world at all!

Stand as the Khalsa, strong as steel, steady as stone;
Give our lives to God and Guru, mind and soul, breath and bone;
Mind and soul are His alone.

The Test of Fire
1980-1984

*A*fter the death of Guru Gobind Singh, the young Sikh nation was beleaguered
and oppressed by the cruel Mugal Governor of Lahore, Zakriya Khan. In 1738,
he arrested Bhai Mani Singh, the pious and learned Head Granthi of the
Golden Temple, for failing to pay an unjustly levied fine. When Bhai Mani Singh was
brought before Zakriya Khan, he was given the sentence of death by torture; to be hacked
alive, limb by limb.

The date was set, the public was gathered, and Bhai Mani Singh was made to sit next
to the bloody chopping block in the public square. A hooded executioner stood over him,
holding a massive sword. As the executioner held Bhai Mani Singh's thumb on the block
preparing to hack it off at the base, Bhai Mani Singh looked up into his face with a steady
gaze.

"Stop!" commanded Bhai Mani Singh, and the executioner cast his cold eyes upon
him. "If you are going to do the job, do it right! This thumb has three joints. Chop it three
ways."

This demand shook the executioner to his bones. What kind of man is this that does not
tremble and pale on the advent of a gruesome death, but welcomes it like a friend! He
dropped his sword and it clattered on the cobblestones. "I ... I can't do that," he stammered.

Bhai Mani Singh said, "Your role is to do your job, and my role is to go through this.
It doesn't matter what the job is, just do it right."

The executioner bowed his head and picked up his sword. He said, "Bhai Sahib, you are a brave man, but may I know just one thing? Why are you doing this? You could have easily paid the fine."

Bhai Mani Singh replied, "The cup of tyranny has become very full. This sacrifice shall be the drop which makes the cup spill over." He closed his eyes, and entered into the peace and bliss of Guru's love as the executioner did his brutal work.

The Sikhs were enraged by the execution of their beloved Bhai Mani Singh, and the persecution that they daily endured. The Khalsa of the Tarana Dal left their homes and took to the jungles of the Lakhi forest. Here they grew strong and waited for the opportunity to strike at the barbarous Mugal Empire so they could once again live free. That opportunity came within months when India was invaded from the north by the armies of Persia, and the Mugal Empire entered its final phase of total collapse.

The Determination to Survive

One morning in the spring of 1980, the Siri Singh Sahib came out from his morning sadhana with tears staining his face. In his meditation he had been struck by a vision of terrible devastation and destruction. He saw an entire generation of young Sikhs lying on the ground, dying in pools of their own blood. The water around the Harimandir Sahib was red from the blood of thousands of Sikhs, and the sky over the Golden Temple churned with black clouds and streaks of lightning. In this vision, death and suffering covered the Sikhs of India like a suffocating blanket of hot ash.

The Sikh Dharma Secretariat immediately sent out a letter to the Sikh leaders in India. "[The Siri Singh Sahib] has shared with us the knowledge that there are only 700 days left for the Sikhs in India to unite and solidify and reorganize; otherwise there will be terrible hardships and great depression for all the brothers and sisters of Sikhism in India.... At that time, there will be like a tidal wave which could overcome the Sikhs. This can be avoided and the future saved by the strength that lies in unity."[1] The letter was virtually ignored.

The Siri Singh Sahib warned the sangat in the West that the decade of the eighties would be fraught with tension, suffering, and bloodshed. He explained that the planet earth was at a time of cusp, the changing of the ages between the Piscean Age and the Age of Aquarius. This was not the first time mankind had faced this trial, and throughout the history of man, these periods of transition were wrenching and destructive.

Difficult days were indeed at hand. The threat of nuclear war was magnified as the cold war between America and the Soviet Union reached new levels of intensity. To add to the gloom of the situation, the possibility of economic collapse in America became an often repeated prediction by the financial sages of the decade. The Siri

Singh Sahib wanted the Khalsa Spiritual Nation to be strong and prepared, not only to merely survive but to serve as an anchor for society.

Sikh Dharma of the Western Hemisphere started contingency planning within their communities. Many people began taking steps to increase their self-sufficiency in case of war or natural disasters such as earthquakes or floods. The Khalsa Council understood its own role in the leadership of the Khalsa Spiritual Nation and allocated resources to developing Ram Das Puri as a place of sanctuary and safety.

The greatest challenge that the Siri Singh Sahib saw in the eighties was the constant assault on the human nervous system that western society was generating. Divorce was at an all-time high, spirits were low, and after the growth years of the sixties, the people of America were slumping into depression and consumerism. In response to this, he began teaching "Survival Yoga, the Art and Science of Surviving the Eighties."

"In the midst of chaos, your greatest ally will be a meditative mind which can stop impulsive behavior and hold you to your basic values; we build this resource in our students through Kundalini Yoga and Raj Yoga. Where love has become distorted and fraudulent, your purest touchstone will be a sense of identity that transcends the confusion of our culture; we build that identity in White Tantric Yoga. In a society where marriages dissolve, a great source of satisfaction and comfort will be your ability to establish and maintain a cozy household that will nurture beautiful children; we teach this through our men's and women's courses. We offer the technology of Healthy, Happy, Holy living. As a network of people committed to righteousness, we extend our support to all people."[2]

That summer he told his students, "The time has come when our steel has to be tested, so let us be ready to temper our steel. Don't hesitate. Die you must. Death shall come to you, but die in Grace. You will never die an ordinary death. One who dies an extraordinary death is a true person in the light of God. Build up your intelligence. Build up your deeds. Build up your personality and your actions."

Ram Das Puri Blooms

In the midst of these survival-minded trends, the development of Ram Das Puri became a high priority. Giant tractor trailers crept up the mountain road loaded with steel girders, and truck after truck of cement wound its way up into the hills. A huge steel pavilion was erected over a 7,000-square-foot cement pad to provide a central area for meditation, meals, and White Tantric Yoga at the Summer Solstice Sadhana camp. Opening out into the Tantric Shelter, a large room was constructed with one wall being a metal rolling door. This was inaugurated as the Sarkar-e-Khalsa Gurdwara, and when the metal wall was rolled up, the entire pavilion was transformed into the Guru's Darbar.

Summer Solstice Sadhana of 1980 brought people from all over the world to celebrate the joyous reunion of the 3HO community on their own land. This year, the tenting site was relocated closer to the Tantric Shelter, making the logistics of meals, children, and evening entertainment less daunting. Another metal building that had been erected the previous year was developed and flush toilets were installed, much to the delight of the many city-born students who attended Solstice. The camp took on a feeling of stability and permanence. It gave the sangat a feeling of security, safety, and pride, knowing that no matter what might be the destiny of the coming years, they would always have a safe place to go.

The Siri Singh Sahib held a vision for the distant future of Ram Das Puri. He foresaw a community of people, highly advanced in matters of spirit, living together, and serving mankind in the radiance of the "Temple of Steel."

"We have started building Guru Ram Das Puri and we intend and hope to gradually finish it. It is a project which will take its own time. It must take planning. It must take endurance. It must come out to be the best in the world! It will be a temple of stainless steel. We have the plan, we have the endurance, and we will build it. We have no doubt about it. It will be a house where our elderly people will come and work as teachers to raise our children, to raise our nation, to pass their days in grace and in tranquillity."[3]

Ram Das Puri is situated in an extraordinary location. Known by the Native Americans to be a place of healing and power, the Pajarito Plateau has always had particular energy properties that enhance the spirit. However, the Siri Singh Sahib

Morning Sadhana at Ram Das Puri

At 3:00 AM, it is very dark in the mountains and sevadars walk between the tents with guitars, singing songs to awaken the campers. Even in June, the early morning air of Ram Das Puri is icy cold, and the temptation to remain curled up in a warm sleeping bag is strong. Slowly the camp comes to life, men, women, and children quietly emerge from their tents and move cautiously in the dark to the cold showers. As they gather together under the Tantric Shelter, the lights from the town of Espanola twinkle in the valley below, competing with the bright stars shining above the silhouette of the mountains. As banis are read, yoga exercises are done, and mantras are chanted, the faint pink of dawn starts its journey across the sky. As the brilliant sun emerges over the crest of the mountain peak, the sangat stands before the Sarkar-e-Khalsa Gurdwara with hands folded in Ardas. The love of this land known as Ram Das Puri seeps in through the pores of the people, and fills the hearts of all the sangat.

perceived something more, and discussed this with the planners and architects of Sikh Dharma. "Due to the energy shifts in the earth's magnetic field, combined with the inclination of the earth's axis now moving into the constellation of Aquarius, Ram Das Puri finds itself situated at a right angle to a cosmic window for the next few thousand years. This means that there will be an enormous increase in energy in this area. The basic purpose of building a temple here in this time and space is to maximize the use of this energy for the purpose of resetting the course of our destiny."[4]

The Temple of Steel was conceived and designed as an ultramodern community and place of prayer for the next millennium. Taking visions of the future and drawing upon the ancient wisdom of the past, the design is overwhelming in concept and scope. The temple itself is the Takhat Raj Yog, crowned by a gigantic double steel arch rising 880 feet into the air that serves to concentrate and magnify the cosmic energy of the Aquarian Age. Surrounding the temple is an impressive 21st century design of marble pavilions, gardens, and housing for a community of young people who will be educated and instructed by the wise teachers and leaders of the future Khalsa Nation.

The Children of the Khalsa

Each summer the children of the Khalsa set up their tents and live upon the high desert of Ram Das Puri. Khalsa Youth Camp was established in 1979 as a spiritual camp to develop healthy bodies, intelligent minds, and God-conscious leaders for the future. The Siri Singh Sahib challenged the camp leaders to "create dependable children, not dependent children."

The routine revolves around the Sikh lifestyle of children's sadhana and gurdwara, nutritious vegetarian meals, and classes in yoga, meditation, Sikh Dharma, and martial arts. There is also plenty of time to enjoy hiking, swimming, camping, arts and crafts, and wilderness skills. The camp fosters the strength in each child to stand up for his or her own beliefs as well as to protect and respect the beliefs of others. The days are very active and well organized, creating self-reliance in the individual, a bond of positive peer support among the children, and trust with the teen and adult guides.

Isolated from the social and chaotic pressures of city life, Khalsa Youth Camp taps the subtle energies of the individual soul. Children are very close to the beautiful and innocent energy of God consciousness, and the expansive and healing environment of Ram Das Puri brings out this delightful quality. The crystal-clean air, pure water, and the unlimited expanse of the western sky open up for the children their undiscovered internal energy.

Normally, the younger age group of three to five year olds are asleep in their tents before dark, as the light remains in the desert summer sky until after 9:00 PM. One night, Camp Director Siri Nam Singh Khalsa, was doing a final check of the tenting area before going to sleep himself. It was a moonless night and exceptionally clear, the expanse of the sky crowded with a multitude of brilliant, blinking stars. He came across a young girl of five sitting quietly outside her tent with her head tilted back, staring at the sky with her mouth open in amazement and delight. He sat down beside her in silence, and together they stared at the sky for a few moments.

She looked at him with wide-eyed excitement and asked, "Where did they all come from?" He realized she had not seen the night sky at Ram Das Puri before because her group was asleep before the stars came out. Before he could answer she whispered in reverent awe, "Is that where God lives?"

"Yes," he answered, "but He also lives inside of you and inside of me." She understood and nodded wisely, tilting her head back again to stare at the sky.

"Children are a gift from God." counseled the Siri Singh Sahib. "We don't own them." The training of camp staff to care for the children keeps this axiom as its guiding principle. Staff are instructed before and throughout camp to foster and nourish the spiritual wonder in each child. One of the teaching tools employed by the camp staff is the "Punjab Puppet Playhouse." Weekly puppet plays are presented to the children to illustrate the values and components of a spiritual lifestyle. **Values cannot be taught, they have to be caught!"** Through the puppet stories, the children have a chance to see spiritual values in action.

Living in the open environment of Ram Das Puri is always a physical challenge, and the absence of the usual social stimuli is a catalyst for mental growth. Hot sun, desert rain showers, and the silent stillness of the desert challenge the tolerance and endurance of the both the staff and the children. The outcome is dramatic, transformational, and always positive. "Letting children stand ruggedly against environments, against chaos, against all, makes them strong. Then children will never be prisoners of their problems, they will be the masters."[5]

Bringing the Traditions West

Guru Gaddee Day, the day the *Siri Guru Granth Sahib* was installed as the last and final Guru of the Sikhs, is a day of festive celebration. When Guru Gobind Singh gave the succession of the Guruship to the *Siri Guru Granth Sahib,* never again would the Khalsa bow their heads to a man. Now the Word of God, the Truth of Truths, prevailed over the Khalsa.

Hacienda de Guru Ram Das in Española had their first Guru Gaddee Day parade in the fall of 1979. The Guru was carried in procession replete with the beat of the drum, the waving of Chauree Sahib, and the sadh sangat vying for the privilege of carrying the *Siri Guru Granth Sahib* on their shoulders. All along the parade route, lights and decorations were laid, and the parade was led by young people swinging and twirling swords in the tradition of gatka. In the years that followed, processions were held all over the West in observance of this great day.

The practice of giving gifts to children, as well as giving gifts of ramalas and decorations to the gurdwara, became an exciting part of the Guru Gaddee Day tradition.

The children looked forward to Guru Gaddee Day with avid anticipation, knowing that a special present wrapped with their name on it could be found lying next to the ramalas in the gurdwara.

In the summer of 1980, Baba Nihal Singh came to the West to visit the summer camps of Sikh Dharma. At KWTC he spoke to the congregation and delivered an enthusiastic message of appreciation for the appearance of the Khalsa in the West. His statuesque appearance and noble demeanor were inspiring and his words were heart-warming. In the Amrit Vela, the sangat sat with him as he recited the daily banis. The western Sikhs learned from his example the correct pronunciation and intonation of the Guru's banis. That summer, Baba Nihal Singh made a recording of his recitation of the daily banis, which still serves today to improve and sharpen their Gurmukhi pronunciation.

On the Siri Singh Sahib's birthday that year, August 26, 1980, the ashrams of the Western Hemisphere celebrated the day by doing a sadhana of two and one-half hours of "Long EkOngKars."[6] It was very nostalgic, remembering the time when that was all the daily sadhana consisted of. They also organized a powerful prayer, channeling the energy of the sangat all over the world. Taking into consideration the time zones, they set an 11-minute simultaneous meditation of the mantra, *Guru Guru Wahe Guru, Guru Ram Das Guru.* In that way the sangats in each country of the world would be chanting at exactly the same time: 4:00 AM in Los Angeles was 12:00 noon in Europe, 9:00 PM in Australia, and so forth around the globe. This mighty prayer for the protection of Guru Ram Das has echoed through the stratosphere every August 26 since then.

Coming to the Feet of Mother India

The violence of 1978 was in brief remission, and the visits to India in the early part of the next decade are remembered as days of innocent inspiration. India was revered as the land where the feet of the Gurus walked, the place where they lived, and where they sat in meditation. India was the motherland. It was the land where the Khalsa was born and where the resplendent Harimandir Sahib stood. In the daily Ardas of the western Khalsa, they prayed with deep sincerity for "a sight and dip in the nectar tank of the Siri Harimandir Sahib."[7]

The tradition of the Unity of Man conference sponsored by the Ruhani Satsang continued, and was again held in New Delhi in February, 1980. The Siri Singh Sahib arrived in New Delhi to speak at the conference in his continuing mission to create trust and cooperation among all religions. He and the jatha arrived shortly after midnight, exhausted from the long flight from Los Angeles. Barely taking time to put the luggage away, the Siri Singh Sahib roused everyone and took them on an ambrosial-hour tour of the historic gurdwaras in Delhi including Sis Ganj, Bangla Sahib, and Rakab Gunj. Sleep was never one of his priorities during these missionary tours, and the people in the yatra struggled to keep up with the pace and intensity of the Siri Singh Sahib's itinerary. When he wasn't at the conference, he set up a reception area in the lobby of the Taj Hotel, seeing all different types of people: dignitaries, friends, and humble Gursikhs.

On September 28, 1980, the sangat traveled to India for their annual yatra. Baba Nihal Singh and his Nihungs escorted the westerners from village to village, doing kirtan, giving speeches, and enjoying the privilege of being in the company of the sadh sangat. The new Guru Ram Das Langar Hall in Amritsar was completed during this time, and Mukia Singh Sahib Guru Terath Singh Khalsa, Chancellor to the Khalsa Council, was the guest speaker at the inaugural celebration. Again, a western jatha played kirtan in Harimandir Sahib on the occasion of Guru Ram Das's birthday. They were feeling the depths of their roots and they established their place in the pulse of life in Amritsar.

The western women were growing impatient, however, with the restrictions placed upon them by the old traditions and customs of the Golden Temple. In general, India was not an enlightened country as to the rights of women and their status in society. But the Siri Singh Sahib had taught them that the status of women in the Khalsa was totally equal to that of men, holding the same rights and responsibilities. If Khalsa was truly without gender, why, they asked, were they not allowed to participate in seva and kirtan at the Golden Temple? Sikh Dharma International formally posed these questions to the Jathedar of the Akal Takhat, Jathedar Gurdial Singh Ajnoha. Through meetings and correspondence they requested greater equality for women in the traditions of the Golden Temple. Acknowledging that the grace and dignity of women must always be maintained, they discussed having days or hours of seva inside the Harimandir Sahib set aside for women only. They requested to be able to play kirtan in the main darbar of the Harimandir Sahib, and to have certain Akand Paths around the parkarma that would be served only by women. They established a deep dialog with the Jathedar, and reached an agreement that progress was to be made, even if only in small steps.

For the Siri Singh Sahib's birthday in 1980, an Akand Path on the roof of the Golden Temple was dedicated for his health and safety. During the bhog ceremony, Vikram Singh Khalsa played kirtan. When he finished he moved to the side, placing the harmonium in front of Krishna Kaur Khalsa and motioned for her to play. A woman had never played kirtan before within the walls of the Harimandir Sahib, and the sevadars started to rise in dark protest of this breach of protocol. But just at that moment, Baba Nihal Singh walked into the sangat with two of his indomitable attendants and bowed before the Guru. He stood and blocked the sevadars' path, and they froze in their tracks, unsure of what to do next. Finally they sat down and Krishna Kaur proceeded with the kirtan. It was joyously concluded with the *Song of the Khalsa* as the morning sun shone through the gurdwara windows.

Meeting of the Sikh Leadership
Even though the political tension in India had lulled, the vision the Siri Singh Sahib had the year earlier still haunted him. He returned to India in January, 1981 for a

meeting with the Sikh leadership to establish a common unity that would serve the Panth Khalsa. Hosted by Baba Nihal Singh in his village of Hakimpur, leaders came from all over India to discuss their commonality and their differences.

Hakimpur is a village deep in the forests of Punjab where Guru Har Rai, the seventh Sikh Guru, camped with his followers for 11 months. Like a place that time had forgotten, Hakimpur preserved the atmosphere and traditions of another age. The gurdwara was grand and rustic, like a medieval fort with massive brick walls, turrets, and a dome top. The village consisted of simple earthen and brick buildings surrounded by forests and fields, with peacocks strolling in the tall grass. Here the Jathedar of Kesgarh Sahib, the President of the Sikh Youth Federation, the President of the S.G.P.C., the President of the Shiromani Akali Dal, the Jathedar of the Dam Dami Takhsal, and many other prominent sevadars of the Panth gathered to discuss their differences and seek a common path of action for the future. Thousands of people came, and the narrow cobblestone streets of the village were alive with activity. There were meetings, speeches, and martial arts presentations by day and kirtan programs each night. Ram Das Kaur Khalsa gave a gatka demonstration, and the Sikhs were astonished to see a woman command with grace the powerful slashing sword. To watch her swinging the sword as Guru Gobind Singh had taught was truly impressive, but even more so was the inspiration she created in the people.

Although there was lengthy dialog among the Sikh leadership, very little common ground was established. The Sikhs were divided, each one intent upon the individual objectives of their own group without seeing the necessity of a consolidated mission.

The Siri Singh Sahib grieved, knowing that the days ahead would be filled with hardship and strife for the Sikhs. When he returned to Amritsar he met with the saintly and respected Baba Karak Singh, a blessed sevadar who worked tirelessly for the construction of gurdwaras in the Punjab. Baba Karak Singh also held the same trepidation for the future of the Khalsa Panth. He foresaw great tragedy looming and asked the western Khalsa to pray for the protection of the Sikhs. He told the Siri Singh Sahib to chant the shabad:

> *Aap sahaaee hoaa sache daa sachaa dhoaa*
> *God himself has come to be my protector, the True One is my only support*

This he explained was a great mantra of protection, vanquishing the enemies of righteousness and dispelling animosity.

Sikh Dharma Foreign Education Program

It was clear that the Sikhs of India needed the fresh inspiration from the West. It was also apparent that the western Khalsa children needed the guidance of India in order to fully understand who they were and from where they had come. This second generation needed to sink their roots in the soil of their Guru, not in the concrete jungle of the technologically advanced but morally bankrupt cities of the West.

"Give me a place where there is no pressure of drugs and sex from the peer group. We want a place where our children can just learn without interference, without prejudice, and without being molested, mentally, spiritually, or physically. We need a spiritual sanctuary for them."[8]

In June, 1981, Dr. Sat Kirpal Kaur Khalsa and Daya Singh Khalsa brought 25 children to India to attend the Guru Nanak Fifth Centenary School (GNFC) in Mussoorie, the school that the Siri Singh Sahib's two younger children, Kulbir Singh and Kamaljit Kaur, had attended. "I am sending these children so that they can grow by themselves with their own grace. They will realize that they can have the courage to go 12,000 miles away and still be who they are. In the future, distance and environments will not matter to them and they will feel our love, protection, and the shield of Guru Ram Das wherever they are."[9]

Their life in India began with living several weeks in Amritsar at the Golden Temple before traveling to Mussoorie. The culture shock for this first group of children was incredible! There was no resemblance between life as they had come to know it, and life in India. Plucked from Saturday morning cartoons and Pizza Hut, they found themselves on an isolated mountain top of the Himalayas. In their view, spirituality was something their parents did, and they didn't see it having much to do with themselves. But now the rules had changed, and their own identity was intricately laced with spiritual growth and endurance.

Nanak Dev Singh Khalsa and Guru Nam Kaur Khalsa were the first American staff to be with the children in 1981, and Gurupreet Singh Khalsa and Gurupreet Kaur Khalsa joined them at GNFC in 1982. The school was run on the principles of the old British Public School system which emphasizes adherence to tight schedules, daily routines, academics, athletics, and hobbies. To this was added the Dharmic practices of the Sikhs: daily recitation of the banis, morning gurdwara, and an emphasis on Sikh History.

The environment was austere and simple. The children lived in dormitories, slept in bunk beds, and kept all their belongings in a wooden cupboard smaller than their toy chests at home. The classrooms were plain and unadorned, without heat or air-conditioning. The playgrounds were open fields, and the children called upon their creativity and imagination to take the place of the intricate electronic games and televisions they had left behind.

The culture shock diminished with time as they were absorbed into the daily routine of school. The environment was free from the drug and sex obsessiveness that was threatening the youth of America and the simple psyche of the beautiful town of Mussoorie pervaded the group. They quickly learned that they were no longer victims of their environments, but masters of it. Their western ways created a healthy cultural exchange, enhancing them as well as their Indian classmates. Deep and meaningful friendships grew between those culturally diverse children.

Every day the western children wore the traditional bana of the Sikhs, and in this they stood alone. "One thing in Sikh Dharma is very unique which you do not understand. It has a tremendous subconscious effect on you. That is the bana which gives you *Niara Panth,* distinct path, which totally pulls you up. There is no way that you can wear this and not be conscious."[10]

Because the school was high in the mountains, they did not have a long summer break, but rather a long winter vacation so that they would not be in the unheated classrooms and dormitories during the season of mountain snow. That first group of children stayed in India during their winter breaks, and most did not return to the United States for more than three years. Throughout this time, many of the children learned to speak Hindi and Punjabi, and to play Gatka and Gurbani Kirtan. Over the months, they discovered personal identity and meaning in the traditions of the Khalsa.

The Nihungs of Baba Nihal Singh

Baba Nihal Singh and his fierce Nihungs accompanied the western boys on a tour in the winter of 1982, giving kirtan and gatka programs in the rural villages of Punjab. Baba Nihal Singh was a role model for the young western boys, casting an image of a true Khalsa man - unmovable dignity, unchallengable strength, and pious devotion. They lived and dressed like Nihungs, riding around the countryside in jeeps with the confident attitude of people who knew who they were and why they were there. As if awakening from amnesia, the boys identified with the Nihung lifestyle in a deep and unfathomable way.

At one gurdwara on the tour, the management did not like Nihungs, and when they heard the group was coming, they closed the iron gates, locking out Baba Nihal Singh and the children. Baba Nihal Singh drove right up to the gates with a jeep full of boys and other Nihungs carrying swords and spears,

as Nihungs always do. With hand movements he beckoned a man inside to come over to the locked gates as if he wanted speak with him. When the man got close, Baba Nihal Singh reached through the bars, grabbed him by the front of his shirt and pulled his face hard into the iron gates. In a deep and menacing voice he demanded that the gates to the gurdwara be unlocked and they be allowed to enter. He explained to him, eyeball to eyeball and nose to nose, that the gates of a gurdwara should never be locked against those who come to bow to the Guru. The man nodded with animation and unlocked the gates without delay. They were served langar and given a graceful place to spend the night. The boys on that trip, who are today grown men with children of their own, tell that story with childish delight, remembering the strength and valor of that Khalsa man who was larger than life - Baba Nihal Singh.

During the winter break of 1982, they went to Amritsar and lived inside the Akal Takhat on the top floor. They woke every morning to the sight and sounds of the Harimandir Sahib right outside their window. They rose and dipped in the nectar tank, and became part of the daily routine of life on the parkarma. These young children, full of mischief and pranks, were accepted and guided by the sevadars of the Golden Temple. They were full of energy, reverent and sometimes irreverent, and they represented and personified the bright future of the Khalsa. Living their life on the parkarma as Sikhs had done for hundreds of years gave these children a solid point of reference that they relied on later in life.

What began as a loose group of parents with children in India transformed into the Sikh Dharma Foreign Education Program under the tutelage of Sardarni Sahiba Dr. Sat Kirpal Kaur Khalsa. By 1983 there were over 100 children participating in the program. Going to school half-way around the world was a difficult thing and a great sacrifice both for the parents and students. But it was soon apparent that the advantages they received were worth the cost. The children developed an intimate bond, a positive peer relationship that supported and guided them. They became self-reliant and developed a mature and secure reasoning with which to measure any situation. As Bhai Daya Singh Khalsa, a ten-year graduate of the SDFE program, put it: "Students educated in the India program are unique in that they learn the limit of their abilities, and the extent of their responsibilities."

Success and Prosperity

From the very beginning, the Siri Singh Sahib guided his people to be financially independent. They needed to build a solid economic foundation, to support themselves and the future of Sikh Dharma of the Western Hemisphere. They needed schools, museums, and hundreds of jobs for the children being born into the Khalsa Nation.

He addressed the Khalsa Council in the spring of 1982, challenging them to rise to the occasion and build this financial base. "Success is a law of infinity. It must come to you all because it is your birthright. The question is, how to create a cycle and how to complete it. We can show how the analytical mind helps to complete the cycle, how the administrative mind helps to retain the cycle, and how the accounting mind can account for everything and make you live in profit. I am grateful and it was my long overdue desire that with this family we would establish ourselves and go ahead with the normal procedure of living successfully."

The Siri Singh Sahib began teaching an extraordinary series of courses on success utilizing the attributes and strengths of people of higher consciousness. In April, 1982, he taught "The Executive Mind"; in 1983, the "Success Cycle Course"; and followed it in 1984 with the course, "Success the Original Way." Joined by other experts in the field, he laid out a basic philosophy and spiritual approach to success and prosperity.

His secret to success he condensed in the following phrase: OPI/OPM. Other People's Intelligence/Other People's Money.

Other People's Intelligence, he explained, is the full utilization of the talents and resources that God has put into your environment. "Your own intelligence cannot solve every problem. Your own intelligence should be applied to how you employ and successfully deploy your environments, your surroundings. That is OPI. Employ and deploy the surroundings. And when you employ the surroundings, don't involve yourself and your ego in it. When you deploy a person, let him use his talent and creativity without impediment. Because it is not *you* in the situation, rather it is your *interest* in the situation. You will get the highest rate of return, because it is not confined to only *you*, your limitations and restrictions. For every person that God brings to your environment, find that person's strength and intelligence and deploy it. That is OPI."

Other People's Money, he explained, is the realization that you have the responsibility to support the grace of your environment. "The money you make is not really yours; 90 percent of it is actually Other People's Money, and it is not yours to spend as you like. This is the law of expansion. Out of every ten dollars, one dollar is mine, and nine dollars are to maintain what is mine. For every one dollar, you require nine dollars to maintain the grace of that one dollar. If you represent yourself with an image that you are ten dollars rich, someone will ask to use it for one hour and you'll give it. Then you'll stand at a bus stop and the driver will not let you on because you don't have a penny! If I make one dollar, I spend only ten cents. When I have ten dollars in my pocket, I know that I actually only have one dollar that is mine, one dollar that is the Guru's and eight dollars that are Other People's Money."

The family businesses were growing and prospering. These companies made a tremendous statement to the public about who and what the people of 3HO were. To a Sikh, work is a form of worship, a spiritual path, and an experience of growth in its own right. These enterprises were and still are, in reality, workshops of consciousness. Growing the businesses of Sikh Dharma meant securing the future of the Khalsa Nation for the generations to come.

The Amrit Bakery in Eugene had become the Golden Temple Bakery, a division of Golden Temple Natural Foods of Oregon, Inc. The bakery had moved to a bigger location, and many hours of labor went into making this building truly a temple. The inside was painted white and pictures of the Gurus and the Golden Temple were placed on the walls. The bakery sound system played Gurbani Kirtan and American Khalsa songs during the day to give the products a high vibration and help the workers keep up. Now the Wha Guru Chews were cooked in large batches in a candy kettle, and the bars were cut and packaged with the help of electric machines instead of being formed by hand in football shapes. More Wha Guru Chews were made in one day than the bakery had previously produced in a month.

In the small rural town of Española, New Mexico, many people had a hard time finding employment. After graduating valedictorian from his police academy class, Singh Sahib Gurutej Singh Khalsa was told he could no longer continue with the police department with his turban and beard because of dress code regulations. On the advice of the Siri Singh Sahib, he and Daya Singh Khalsa formed their own security company, Akal Security, Inc. Based on high standards of training and innovative management, Akal Security grew rapidly throughout the State of New Mexico. The word *akal* means "without death," and was the traditional cry of the Sikhs when charging into battle. Their distinctive uniform of khaki with a navy blue turban and neckscarf was outstanding and soon became a well-known trademark. Their natural instincts as soldier/saints were complemented by state-of-the-art training and the men of Akal Security quickly earned the reputation of courage under fire. The company motto of Akal Security was "In God We Trust." As Gurutej Singh explained, "When we wear that uniform into the night, we never know what we will have to deal with. Things can change in an instant. We can only remember that 'In God we trust.'"

Siblings of Destiny

In the Khalsa Council meetings of January, 1983, the Siri Singh Sahib expressed his impatience with the development of the Sikhs in the West. There was so much to do, and so little time in which to do it. He challenged the Khalsa Council to take the leadership and to recognize and fulfill their responsibility as "Siblings of Destiny."

"We who are the siblings of the soul, why are we wasting time? We have the destiny, better that we fill it. We have the dignity, better that we live it. We have the divinity, better that we share it. We have the grace, better that we spread it. You are the siblings of the spirit. You are the siblings of the soul. You are the Siblings of Destiny.

"Understand that we have four difficult years before us, 1984 to 1988. I have a sensitivity that we will come through it, but if not, we will be the only remnants left to tell the story. Simply, you must not fail in keeping up. Keep going and you will reach the destination. Stop for nothing. The work has just begun. Let us do it forever so that we can experience the truth of these lines:

> *Jinee naam dhiaaiaa gae mashakat ghaal,*
> *Naanak te mukh ujale,*
> *Ketee chhutee naal.*

> *Those who have meditated on the Name and departed having*
> *worked very hard, Nanak, their faces are radiant and many are*
> *freed along with them.*
>
> Guru Nanak, Japji Sahib

As mother earth rotates and father sun shines, we will meet our destiny, because we are the Siblings of Destiny."[11]

In May, 1983, Sikh Dharma mourned the death of Sardar Hukam Singh. His passing was a great loss to the western Sikhs as he had provided the Sikh Dharma Secretariat with more than ten years of inspiration, friendship, and guidance. He had become a tutor to those striving to develop and nourish the delicate relationship between east and west. He gently but firmly smoothed off the rough edges of their American bluntness in speech, and counseled them on the intricacies of the oriental mind. As an honest and impartial mentor, his guidance was often sought and relied upon, and he never betrayed the trust that was given him. During his years in service to India, he was the Governor of Rajisthan in the early 1970s, a Member of Parliament, and served also as a Speaker of the Indian Parliament (Lok Subha). He founded the *Spokesman* newspaper and served as its editor for many years, so his advice in political perspective was impeccable. As Sikh Dharma of the Western Hemisphere entered the difficult days that lay ahead, his counsel and advise was acutely missed.

The Science of Naad

In 1980, the Siri Singh Sahib received his Doctorate of Psychology in the field of communication. His thesis paper, entitled "Communication - Liberation or Condemnation" opened new doors on the topic of human intercommunication. Drawing upon his extensive knowledge of *Naad,* the science of sound and communication, he brought into modern context the ancient teaching of this science.

During the Khalsa Women's Training Camp of 1983, the Siri Singh Sahib lectured on "The Psychology of the Invincible Woman." In his lectures and yoga classes, he revealed secrets of the sound current inherent in the banis, creating a deep understanding of the Sikh technologies. The women bowed with synchronicity to the beat of Jaap Sahib sung with harmonium and tabla, experiencing the science of Naad and Gurbani.

"Naad means 'the essence of all sounds.' All languages contain sounds which relate to one or more of the five elements of air, fire, water, earth, or ether. Gurbani is the perfect combination and permutation of sounds relating to all the five elements in complete balance. When Guru Arjun Dev, the fifth Guru Nanak, compiled the *Siri Guru Granth Sahib,* in 1604, he only included those banis which were in Naad. These compositions are called Gurbani.

"There are eighty-four meridian points on the upper palate of a human's mouth. One can feel that upper palate with the tongue and experience its different surfaces. There are two rows of meridian points on the upper palate and on the gum behind the upper teeth. The tongue stimulates those meridian points, and they in turn stimulate the hypothalamus which makes the pineal gland radiate. When the pineal gland radiates, it creates an impulsation in the pituitary gland. When the pituitary gland gives impulsation, the entire glandular system secretes and a human being obtains bliss. This is the science.

"The whole language of Gurbani has the power to make a person divine, just in its recitation, if done correctly. One need not be concerned with the meaning for a change in consciousness. Bani has to be understood by the heart, not by the head.

There is no power in the head, it is in the heart. The head is for God and the heart is for you. That is why Guru Gobind Singh asked for the head, and not for the heart. Whosoever lives with the head to God and heart for self, that prayer is complete."[12]

For the first time since KWTC had begun eight years before, the Siri Singh Sahib personally taught Kundalini Yoga exercises daily. He pushed his students harder and harder, building their strength of heart, mind, and body for the trials he knew lay ahead.

"A first-rate teacher is a teacher who is very hard, very intolerant of the mistakes of the students, and he gives a crushing blow on every step. This is first rate. A second rate teacher is one who just reminds a person of his mistakes, and a third rate teacher is one who just pleases him. The harder the teacher is, the better one can learn; the softer the teacher is, the less one can learn. Because all the time you are in a fight between the ego and the soul, the conscious and unconscious mind.

"The job of the teacher is to give you the most impossible work. And the job of the student is to do it. And, mind you, it may be a total loss. But you are going to develop the power to make the impossible become possible. And when a person under pressure can develop a consciousness that he can make the impossible to become possible, he is perfect! Give a student an impossible job. If he does it, then give him two more. If he does it, give him six! Eight! *Ten!*"[13]

He left KWTC in August to attend the annual European Yoga Festival in the south of France. There were now over 60 teachers in Europe, and this event was a time of reunion, communion, and rejuvenation for more than 300 students.

During this tour, and many times to follow, the Siri Singh Sahib visited Pope John Paul II in Rome. Each acknowledged that man's only hope lay in the power of prayer, and offered prayers for each other and the struggles of their people.

The Peace in Punjab is Broken

Political events in India had become ridden with strife and violence throughout 1983, and the peaceful life in Amritsar had radically and forever changed. The Sikhs in the West struggled to understand the increasing volatility of the situation. It was a great act of faith and courage for parents to send their children to India, 12,000 miles away from home, when there were so many unanswered questions.

The Siri Singh Sahib traveled to India in January, 1984, and encouraged as many people as possible to join him. He warned them that the time might come when they couldn't visit the Harimandir Sahib, and they should take the opportunity to do so now. But for the most part his words fell on deaf ears. No one could even dream of a situation where the western Sikhs would be denied the chance to go and meditate at the Golden Temple. It had become such an essential and routine part of their lives.

When the children visited the Harimandir Sahib during the winter break of 1983, they could no longer stay in the Akal Takhat. The Dam Dami Takhsal had set up an armed camp there, and no one was allowed to enter the upper floors. The Babbar Khalsa[14] had similarly occupied the top floor of Guru Nanak Nivas, so no longer could the students feel at home and relaxed within the Golden Temple complex. Narinderjit Singh the Information Officer of the Golden Temple was always there for the staff and the children, protecting and guiding them. That winter the children stayed in other gurdwaras in Punjab, away from the troubles of Amritsar.

The morchas[15] had begun, and huge groups of Sikhs in orange turbans offered themselves for arrest daily in peaceful protest against the central government in Delhi. There was little that made sense in the heightening violence and animosity between the Sikhs and Hindus. The western Sikhs didn't comprehend the depth of the situation, but neither did most of their Indian friends who lived and worked in Amritsar. From the Americans' standpoint, the Sikh demands seemed to be straightforward issues where a minority people were seeking to gain their rights with regard to religious expression in their home state of Punjab. The problem appeared to be all in the political maneuvering, which reached beyond the scope of the Sikh demands.

One thing that was clearly understood was the feeling of electric tension and imminent danger. Guns and other weapons were visible everywhere and the city had begun to take on the look and feel of an armed military camp. The western Sikhs did not know when they left Amritsar in the spring of 1984 that they would not see the Harimandir Sahib again for six long, dreadful years.

The Year of the Guru

In the January, 1984 Khalsa Council meetings, the Siri Singh Sahib declared 1984 to be "The Year of the Guru."

"Chauraasee, eighty-four, is what the karma is. This is the year of liberation and solidarity, intelligence and consciousness; and so we declare it as the Year of the Guru. We are entering 1984, a well defined planetary year in which the spirit shall prevail and excel. Also, it will be test of the time."[16]

Unlike other religious writings, the *Siri Guru Granth Sahib* is not the history of a people or a religion. It is not a scripture. It is the experience of the soul, and its journey through life to the Oneness of God. The *Siri Guru Granth Sahib* is what gives a Sikh the experience of his higher nature. For the Sikh, the *Siri Guru Granth Sahib* is not a book, it is the supreme living wisdom that removes ignorance through its Truth and through the repetition of its powerful sound current.

"It is very beautiful that I have Guru as my friend, and my friend shall continue to be Guru. And that is the only relationship which I seek, and I shall seek, the Word of Truth. The Word I worship and to the Word I bow. The Word I remember and the Word I chant. The Word is all my life is. My beginning, my now, and my end is the Word."[17]

Gur bin ghor andhaar,
Guru bin samajh naa aavai.
Gur bin surat naa sidh,
Guru bin mukhat naa paavai.

Without the Guru, there is pitch darkness
And without the Guru, understanding is not obtained.
Without the Guru, mystical experience and spiritual power is not possible,
And without the Guru, one cannot be liberated.

Siri Guru Granth Sahib Ji, pg. 1399

Resolution of the Khalsa Council

*W*hereas, the Khalsa Council serves to determine policy and guidelines for the growth of the Khalsa nation as the representative body of the sadh sangat, and

Whereas, the Khalsa Council is a nation which is a state of consciousness which pulls people of consciousness together to work for the common goal of living for each other, as the siblings of destiny,

And the year 1984 being the year of the 84th cycle of the twentieth century, a number which represents the opportunity to transcend the pain and duality of the world through the power of prayer,

Recognizing that the Guru is the Word of Truth and this Word is the begin-

ning, the end and the present, the Word is what we worship, to the Word we bow, the Word we chant and the Word is our entire life,

And having acknowledged that our friend is Guru and our friend shall continue to be Guru and that being the only relationship which we seek,

Recognizing that the Dharma is established by the Will of God and through the Grace of Guru, and it is the destiny of the planet earth in which the birth of Khalsa shall be celebrated and will expand, grow and establish the rule of Truth,

We hereby resolve that the year 1984 shall be observed as the Year of the Guru.

The Martyrdom of the Akal Takhat

On June 6, 1984, the Indian Army invaded the Golden Temple, destroying the Akal Takhat, the museum, the historical library, and many other buildings within the complex. Military tanks rolled onto the marble parkarma and the holy and historical Akal Takhat, built by the hands of Guru Hargobind, was attacked by mortar rockets. Thousands of Sikhs were killed in the attack, both peaceful pilgrims and armed defenders. Rivers of blood flowed on the parkarma and the life of every Sikh was changed forever.

The devastating news of the June 6 invasion of the Harimandir Sahib by the Indian Army struck the western Khalsa, as it did Sikhs all over the world, like a deep knife wound. The Harimandir Sahib and the Sikhs of the Punjab were bound to the heart center of the western Sikhs, and as the horrifying stories came leaking out of Amritsar, hearts all over the world were broken. Copious tears flowed as people wept in disbelief, in shock, in denial, in grief, and in anger. Prayers were offered, but the news turned from bad to worse and it seemed to some that God had turned His face away from the suffering of the Khalsa Nation.

"There is nothing which could happen that is more damaging to the whole of humanity than what has been done in this last week. This doesn't hurt just the Sikhs, don't misunderstand! What has been done to the Sikhs has been done to the entire humanity. The psyche of the world has been totally shaken. The peace of the world has been shattered. Throughout history whenever the Harimandir Sahib has been desecrated, dynasties fell. Try to understand the coincidence of the psycho-magnetic field in the interpretation of the magnetic light of lights which governs and revolved this earth. See what is happening and what is being done and to what extent. It is shocking!"[18]

The Siri Singh Sahib called a conference in Santa Fe, New Mexico on June 23, 24, and 25. Leaders from England, Malaysia, Singapore, and the United States came to discuss the situation and share their sorrow and pain. The horrible act of desecration of the Harimandir Sahib and the multitude of lives lost created in each Sikh a strong determination and rebirth into his own strength of faith. From the meeting emerged a basic policy of unity. They established goals that included the restoration of basic civil liberties and human rights for the Sikhs of Punjab. One of their main thrusts was to make sure that the world was informed and this horror would not remain hidden behind a wall of secrecy.

"This is not a time to become emotional or angry. It is a time to act. If we can share this pain with the world at large, we will carry the day. Every person, every newspaper, television, radio station shall share our pain. Fourteen million Sikhs are under siege. It is a war of identity of people who love God and feel God within them. If we in the West can create environments to let the people know that it is a matter of human identity, we'll carry the entire West with us."[19]

Sikh Dharma International printed a detailed brochure on the "Martyrdom of the Akal Takhat" and distributed it widely. They talked extensively on radio and television, printed articles, and protested the military action in India through every means possible. To pray for the millions of Sikhs suffering under tyranny and persecution in Punjab, the ashrams across the world started a special evening meditation that included the shabad: *Aap sahaaee hoaa sache daa sachaa doaa, Har, Har, Har.* The next year it was included in their morning sadhana routine.

Sikhs are not strangers to sacrifice, and throughout history they have stood that ultimate test of faith. The Siri Singh Sahib counseled his people that even this horrible event had to be, by the nature its existence, within the Will of God. The Akal Takhat stood in smoldering ruins, burned and broken by mortar and tank shells. But what force on earth had the power to vanquish such a seat of spiritual and temporal authority? None. Surely not that of the Indian Army. So, like Guru Teg Bahadur and Guru Arjun Dev, the Akal Takhat had voluntarily offered itself for sacrifice, in the Name of *Akal Purkh*, the Undying One, for the victory of the Sikh people.

"A human can make a sacrifice, but sometimes that is not enough. The Akal Takhat has its own independent sovereign identity, and it has reached its own martyrdom. I, as a Sikh, have no right to question why the Akal Takhat did what it did. If I question, then I am not a Sikh of the Guru. But I know that there is no power on earth so strong that they could destroy the Akal Takhat unless the Akal Takhat chose to give itself as a sacrifice.

"There is no history of mankind where a sacrifice has been made and the nation has not become victorious. Guru Arjun gave the sacrifice and we became victorious. Guru Teg Bahadur gave the sacrifice, and we became victorious. Guru Gobind Singh's entire family gave the sacrifice and we became victorious. Today, our Akal Takhat has chosen to offer itself as a sacrifice, and we shall not lose.

"Akal Takhat wanted at this moment to awaken the Khalsa nation. This nation could not have been awakened with any sacrifice less. People who have never chanted Japji in their whole life are now rising in the morning to pray. What sacrifice other than the Akal Takhat could have awakened them? I think that God has said to Akal Takhat 'Go ahead now. Sacrifice. It is very timely. It will awaken every sleeping soul.'

"The time is very hard and we have been hit harshly. I know that if the Akal Takhat chose to give itself as a sacrifice, then it must be required. To awaken the Sikhs, there was no other way. That has been done now. The nation will wake up, will rise in spirit and will win. It is the greatest sacrifice to ever be made. It will bring the greatest result that could ever have been encashed."[20]

1984—The Year of Death and Destruction

On October 31, 1984, Prime Minister Indira Gandhi was assassinated, allegedly shot to death by her Sikh bodyguards at her home in New Delhi. With planned precision, riots almost immediately erupted in Delhi and all over India with Hindus seeking bloody retribution against Sikhs. With the news of an estimated 10,000 people dead in New Delhi alone reaching the wire services, the parents whose children were studying in India waited with patience and faith to hear news from Mussoorie. Nearly all contact had been lost with India and there were grave concerns for the safety of the 150 western Sikh students. It was a time when the heart of every mother and father of Sikh Dharma was laid bare on the altar of faith.

In the town of Mussoorie, tensions ran high. Outsiders had come into town to incite the local people and create disorder. There was rioting, and Sikh businesses and properties were attacked and burned throughout Mussoorie and the Doon Valley. That night, Gurupreet Singh and Nanak Dev Singh stayed at Shangri-La, the girl's campus, alert and on guard with swords in hand. The Indo-Tibetian Border Police had a training center near the school, and they were alerted and placed on stand-by to be deployed if the situation worsened. But the night passed without incident, and with time, Mussoorie returned to its normal pace of life.

This was not true for the rest of India. After a few weeks, Gurupreet Singh and Nanak Dev Singh went down the mountain to visit the gurdwara at Paonta Sahib to check on their friends there. As soon as they left the isolated town of Mussoorie, they felt the horrible weight of fear and discrimination that had descended upon the Sikhs of India as the army continued its pursuit of Sikh "activists." Pulling them off the bus, the police interrogated them along with anyone else with beard and turban. India, the motherland, had suddenly become a hostile stranger.

Dr. Sat Kirpal Kaur Khalsa visited India in December, shortly after the riots, to attend to the business of Sikh Dharma Foreign Education. Signs of death and destruction were everywhere in New Delhi and the Sikh community was still reeling with shock and fear. People didn't know if they would again be pulled from their beds, tortured and burned alive in the streets. They were shattered. Bangla Sahib Gurdwara, usually a hub of devotion and activity, was nearly empty for Asa di Var in the morning, as only a handful ventured out of their homes in the dark.

After years of traveling to India, when Dr. Sat Kirpal Kaur received her visa this time it bore a new stamp that read: "Not valid for restricted and protected areas." The borders of Punjab were sealed, and despite all efforts she was denied permission to visit the Golden Temple. Martial law had descended and a news blackout prevailed. Precious little information was available and the western Khalsa could not determine the status of their friends, whether they lived or had died. They were foreigners in the land they had come to regard as their spiritual home.

Notes

1. Shakti Parwha Kaur Khalsa in a letter to Sikh leaders, January 7, 1980
2. Yogi Bhajan; *The Yoga Journal*, Jan/Feb. 1980
3. Yogi Bhajan; *Beads of Truth*, Dec. 1980
4. Guruhans Singh Khalsa; *Beads of Truth*, December 1980
5. Yogi Bhajan; Khalsa Council, Winter 1982
6. *Ek Ong Kar Sat Nam Siri Wahe Guru* chanted in a specific meter and breath
7. English translation of the daily Ardas or prayer of the Sikhs
8. Yogi Bhajan; Khalsa Council, Winter 1982
9. Bhajan Yogi; lecture December 13, 1987
10. Yogi Bhajan; *Beads of Truth*, Summer 1985
11. Yogi Bhajan; *Siblings of Destiny,* Khalsa Council 1983
12. Yogi Bhajan; *Psyche of the Soul,* Handmade Books 1993
13. Yogi Bhajan, Khalsa Women's Training Camp lecture, 1983
14. The Dam Dami Taksal and the Babbar Khalsa are different Sikh groups in India.
15. In peaceful defiance of the government's ban on group assembly, the morchas were large, organized gatherings of people willingly courting arrest, filling up the jails night after night, in order to draw attention to their legitimate demands.
16. Yogi Bhajan; *Beads of Truth,* Summer 1984
17. Bhajan Yogi, *Beads of Truth*, Summer 1984
18. Bhajan Yogi, Gurdwara lecture, June 11, 1984
19. Yogi Bhajan; Sikh Religious Conference, June 28, 1984
20. Yogi Bhajan, Gurdwara lecture, July 1, 1984

When Will I Walk on the Cold Marble Again?

by S.S. Guru Das Singh Khalsa

When will I walk on the cold marble again?
When will I feel the golden light in my eyes?
Bathe in the holy waters. Dress your altar with flowers.
When will I walk on the cold marble again?

The silence of death has killed the song so ageless,
The turning of the pages, the prayers of the pure.
The waters turn red, the sky above has darkened.
Amidst these walls of silence, our prayers can be heard.

The Earth cries in pain, her heart has been broken,
Her sons have been stolen, imprisoned, and slain.
And those who remain, their spirit grows stronger.
They suffer no longer, sheltered in the Name.

We shall rise again, in grace and strength together.
We'll sing our song forever and righteousness will reign.
The banner of the Name will wave in skies of glory.
As time will write our story, we sing "never again."

Soon we will walk on the cold marble again.
Soon we will feel the golden light in our eyes.
Bathe in the holy waters. Dress your altar with flowers.
Soon we will walk on the cold marble again.

Chapter Five

Hail Guru Ram Das and Heal the World 1985-1994

*O*ne day Mansa Devi, the saintly wife of Guru Amar Das, came with folded hands before the Guru. "Oh husband," she implored, "the time has come for our daughter, Bibi Bani, to be married. Can you, in your exalted being, choose for her a husband?"

Guru Amar Das said, "Of course. What kind of boy are you asking for?"

"He must be a devoted Sikh from a good family," replied Mataji. "He should be respectful and serviceful, humble and yet strong of heart. And his features should reflect the beauty of his inner nature."

As she spoke, she looked out the window and saw a young man walking along the street selling boiled wheatberries. He was an orphan, dressed in ragged clothes, but his face glowed with an inner light that came from a blessed soul. Pointing him out to her husband she said, "Like him. Let us find a young man like that for Bibi Bani."

Guru Amar Das sent his personal attendant to fetch the boy. The attendant went out and said, "Come with me. The Guru wishes to see you."

The boy shook with fear and said, "Did I do something wrong? Did I shout too loudly? Please forgive me and tell the great Guru that I will never do that again!"

Finally the boy was persuaded to come before the Guru. The Guru said, "Mataji, please look at this boy, radiant with God's love. Is this what you mean?"

"Yes, yes!" she replied, "A boy just like him would be suitable to marry our daughter."

The Guru said, "Well, now, if the boy you search for is to be just like him, then it shall be him. In all of this world and the next there is not another being like him. He is unparalleled. We need search no further for he alone is suitable to marry Bibi Bani."

Through his devotion to the one God and his pure love for Guru Amar Das, the poor orphan boy named Jetha married Bibi Bani. He rose to become Guru Ram Das, the forth Guru of the Sikhs and the only one to sit on the throne of Raj Yog. That a poor orphan boy could have this exalted destiny is the miracle of Guru Ram Das.

Dhan dhan Raam Daas Gur, Jin siriaa tinai savaariaa.

Pooree hoee karaamaat, aap sirjanhaarai dhaariaa.

Honored and praised is Guru Ram Das,

the One who created You has adorned You.

Perfect is Your miracle,

The Creator Himself has installed You on the Throne.[1]

Prayers for the Punjab

The dawn of 1985 brought with it searing reports from India. The Indian military moved through the rural districts of Punjab, routing out political dissention with savage brutality. The scant information coming out of Punjab was very grim as a campaign against the Sikh youth was in full swing. Before the violence began to subside, upwards of 100,000 people had been killed. The Khalsa of the West mourned the devastation of their people and their spiritual home.

"Do you know what happened in the Punjab? The young people got excited, wound up, but no one prepared them. Now, a block of one age group is totally eliminated. A link from the page of history has been taken away. If communism has succeeded anywhere, it has succeeded among Sikhs. They took our youthful bud of intelligentsia and put it to death. And that is how unprepared, unsecular, and without understanding we were in Punjab. Now with lawsuits and blackmail they are even trying to force me to agree with their dirty schemes, but I will not.

"It is not only that one hundred thousand people have just died. An age group that had the most vital link in the history of this Dharma has been eliminated forever. There's nobody left to tell the story. Instead of using these one hundred thousand people all over the world to spread the Word of the Guru, they have been put before bullets. It was a most organized crime, and it was done with coldness and calculation.

"Those who call themselves Sikhs, who are butchering young Sikhs and being paid with communist money, shall ultimately lose. It is the biggest plot of this time, to prevent the Sikhs from uniting. People are being bought and sold like potatoes."[2]

Prevented from entering the Punjab, the sangat longed in vain to go to Amritsar and offer whatever they could to ease the pain of the Khalsa Panth. This was not possible on any level, and many wrung their hands under the heavy weight of enforced inaction. News filtered to the West that the Akal Takhat had been rebuilt by the Indian government, and the Sikhs in India had torn it down in protest. The sangat of the West was stunned and they wanted to build the Akal Takhat with their own hands. Since they couldn't enter the Punjab, this was out of the question. So instead they rebuilt the Akal Takhat the only way they could—through prayer and meditation.

"Akal Takhat is not brick and mortar, hands and money, government and bombardment, or destruction and construction. That is not Akal Takhat. The Akal Takhat is the nerve center of the universe that keeps the central rotation of the magnetic shield of the planet. They have damaged that place, and they do not know what they have done. They thought it was a building. They thought there were some people hiding, and they thought they could bombard it and kill it. And then they thought they could bring the artisans, and bring some marble, and some gold, and they could rebuild it. If Akal Takhat could be built like that, then we could have Akal Takhat clones everywhere. We could have two million Akal Takhats. They don't realize that a body can have two lungs, but it can only have one heart.

"Akal Takhat cannot be built by governments. Guru Arjun has to sit again through the test of fire as Khalsa, and we shall chant the mantra that he chanted to purify himself. That is what the *Naaraain Shabad* is. We shall sing this shabad to participate in the full glory of it. We are Sikhs of the shabad, and we are sons and daughters of Guru Gobind Singh.

"You shall build the Akal Takhat. Each line of this shabad is a brick. Each breath that goes with the shabad is the gold. And each voice that creates it is the marble. We shall construct the Akal Takhat with the power of the shabad."[3]

The sangat of Sikh Dharma of the Western Hemisphere started a tradition, which continues today, of Gurdwara programs in honor of the Akal Takhat on the sixth day of every month. Together they meditated and prayed for the young Sikhs who were suffering the pain of torture and unjust incarceration. They sang the Naaraain Shabad with a deep prayer as they projected their spiritual selves with sincerity into the kar seva of rebuilding the Akal Takhat.

The sorrow and heartbreak of the situation in Punjab had far-reaching and devastating effects. The Siri Singh Sahib became ill. His face was ashen and his blood pressure soared. It was obvious that the pressure of these tragic times was exacting a heavy toll on him as it was on every Sikh leader. The doctors told him he had to slow down, reduce his travel schedule, and minimize the stress in his environment. Because White Tantric Yoga has a consuming effect on the Mahan Tantric, the course was changed to a one-day format to minimize the stress on his body. Entitled "Life Force Experience," the new one-day course was well received by the 3HO students. Still he would not slow the pace or the tempo of his life. All day was spent dealing with the

Naaraain, Naaraain

The Name of the Immaculate Lord is Ambrosial Water. Chanting it with the tongue, sins are washed away.

Naam niranjan neer Naraain
Rasanaa simrat paap bilaain.

The Lord abides in everyone. The Lord illumines each and every heart. Chanting the Lord's Name, the mortal does not fall into hell. Serving the Lord, all fruitful rewards are obtained.

Naaraain sabh maaeh nivaas
Naaraain ghat ghat pargaas
Naaraain kehtay narak na jaaeh
Naaraain sayv sagal fal paaeh

Within my mind is the Support of the Lord. The Lord is the boat to cross over the world-ocean. Chanting the Lord's Name, the Messenger of Death runs away. The Lord breaks the teeth of Maya, the witch.

Naaraain man maaeh adhaar
Naaraain bohith sansaar
Naaraain keht jam bhaag palaain
Naaraain dant bhaanay daain

The Lord is forever and ever the Forgiver. The Lord blesses us with peace and bliss. The Lord has revealed His Glory. The Lord is the mother and father of His Saint.

Naaraain sad sad bakhshind
Naaraain keenay sookh anand
Naaraain pragat keeno partaap
Naaraain sant ko maaee baap

The Lord, the Lord, is in the Sadh Sangat, the Company of the Holy. Time and time again, I sing the Lord's Praises. Meeting with the Guru, I have attained the Incomprehensible Object. Nanak the slave, has grasped the Support of the Lord.

Naaraain saadh sang Naraain
Baarambaar Naraain gaain
Basat agochar gur mil lehee
Naaraain ot Naanak daas gehee

problems of Sikh Dharma of the Western Hemisphere, and all night was spent on the telephone dealing with the problems in India. In the dire atmosphere of the times, there was no opportunity to lessen the load.

The West Prays for Peace

As he traveled across the United States, Canada, and Europe teaching the "Life Force Experience" course, the Siri Singh Sahib set up meetings in each city with the local religious leaders. He focused his attention on establishing communication and cooperation among the various religions and spiritual groups. One consistent theme he stressed in all his meetings and lectures was to pray for world peace and to never underestimate the power of prayer! Following his lead, ashrams throughout the world became active participants in local interreligious councils and activities.

Understanding that peace comes through prayer, the Siri Singh Sahib inaugurated "Peace Prayer Day" at Ram Das Puri in June, 1985. In what was to become an annual event of the 3HO Foundation, people gathered from all over the world to share this day of prayer on the beautiful mountain site of Ram Das Puri in New Mexico. Over 2,000 people attended including representatives from all major faiths, politicians, friends, and students. Together they prayed for world peace, for peace in India, and for peace in each individual soul. "When the prayer for peace encircles the entire globe," said the Siri Singh Sahib, "only then will this planet be united as one."

Paying the Price of Stress

Refusing to yield to the wishes of his doctors that he reduce his tempo of life, the health of the Siri Singh Sahib continued to decline. In September, 1986, he underwent an angioplasty procedure in an attempt to forestall the progression of heart disease. As a result the Siri Singh Sahib was forced to suspend his traveling and teaching schedule. His unrelenting pace over the past 18 years of teaching, traveling, and counseling without taking the time to care for himself physically had levied a heavy toll. Finally his body rebelled, stating loud and clear: STOP!

"There is a disease that I am a victim of, and that I have inflicted on myself. It is called STRESS. When the Golden Temple was attacked, I lost my yogiship. I cried in gurdwara when I stood to speak. A yogi is supposed to be able to control the emotions. This stress is not going to go down. It is going to go up and up."[4]

The aftermath of the procedure required him to adhere to a very strict diet and participate in intense cardiovascular rehabilitation. Dr. Soram Singh Khalsa, who has a flourishing medical practice in Beverly Hills, served as the Siri Singh Sahib's personal doctor, monitoring his many medicines, herbs, and supplements.

Dr. Alan Singh Weiss, without thought for his own privacy or comfort, opened his home to the Siri Singh Sahib, providing a graceful environment for him in which to rest and heal. Siri Simran Kaur Khalsa, who became Alan's wife in February, 1987, served as medical attendant to the Siri Singh Sahib, monitoring his food, administering his medication, and doing her best to limit visitors. They still serve in those roles today, and the selfless sacrifice of their personal lives to the recovery of the Siri Singh Sahib's health is a debt the sangat will never be able to repay.

Still the process of heart disease was not arrested, and in December, 1986, the Siri Singh Sahib underwent a second angioplasty procedure. True to his nature, every time he started to recover and regain some of his energy and metabolic momentum, he would again pick up the pace of the schedule and submit to the constant demands for his time and attention. The needs were so great and the solutions so difficult that even his capable staff was not able to restrict his constant involvement. In July of 1993, he underwent triple bypass heart surgery and after a brief period of recovery, picked up his schedule again.

The plight of the sangat in India affected the health of many other Sikh leaders around the world as well. In England, journalist Singh Sahib Gurcharn Singh Khalsa suffered a deep anguish since the invasion of the Golden Temple in 1984. He was a beloved friend of the Siri Singh Sahib and an admired and respected brother of the sangat. He had frequently visited America, encouraging and actively participating in the Khalsa Council meetings. A true Sikh of the Guru, he never saw the difference between an Indian, American, or African Sikh. He always maintained his dedication and love for the ideals of Guru Gobind Singh, and throughout his life was an example of those very ideals. He died in the fall of 1987, much to the sorrow of the western sangat.

The Sangat Carries the Load

For the first time since the formation of 3HO in 1969, the Siri Singh Sahib did not attend Winter Solstice in December, 1986. For many years the Siri Singh Sahib had been explaining the importance of gathering together to build the strength of group consciousness, and now without his presence the reality of that became very clear. More than ever Winter Solstice served to renew the sangat, uplifting their spirits and inspiring their faith. Powerful prayers for the rapid healing of the Siri Singh Sahib were offered as once again the sangat turned to the power of meditation in a time of crisis.

Now that the Siri Singh Sahib's health would not allow him to travel, plans were underway for a new format of White Tantric Yoga. Under the Siri Singh Sahib's direction videotaped kriyas and mantras were prepared and produced by Sat Simran Kaur Khalsa. The new course format was titled "Renew to be New." This allowed the Mahan Tantric to meditate at home in his own environment, processing and filtering the tantric energy through his subtle body while the participants performed the kriyas in their cities according to his pre-recorded direction.

The students of 3HO Foundation were slow to embrace this new format. They longed for the actual presence of the Siri Singh Sahib, to hear him speak and to seek his counsel on their personal questions. More than anything else the physical absence of the Siri Singh Sahib at the "Renew to Be New" courses made them face the reality that one day the Siri Singh Sahib would not be on the physical plane of the earth. How-ever, as they participated more and more in the new format of White Tantric Yoga, it became clear that the dynamic energy of the tantric meditation was still very much present. The meditation took on a deeper, more mature quality.

Planning Summer Solstice Sadhana, 1987 was a great challenge not knowing if the Siri Singh Sahib would be physically present. Solstice was started without him and the sangat worked together to make the camp a dynamic success.

Three days of "Renew to Be New" videotaped meditations were held for the first time at a Solstice gathering in the absence of the Siri Singh Sahib. As is customary, the last day of the White Tantric Yoga meditations was the "blind walk." Hand in hand, strings of ten to fifteen people with their eyes closed and their minds concentrated in meditation were guided by a leader through the fields of Ram Das Puri in a blind, walk-ing meditation. Looking out on the green fields, 100 lines of white-dressed people could be seen weaving through the tall grass, chanting God's name. At the end of the meditation, all the lines were guided blindly past the Tantric Shelter to an area in front of the Siri Singh Sahib's cabin. As the meditation came to an end, the group inhaled..., exhaled..., and opened their eyes. There before them stood the Siri Singh Sahib on his porch with his arms open wide. The stunned silence soon erupted into cries of joy! The sangat was profoundly grateful to see him and their outpouring of love created an emotion-filled reunion.

Peace Prayer Day, 1987 was guided by a heartfelt offering of prayer. The highlight was when the Flame of Peace was carried by marathon runners from its home at the Sanctuario de Chimayo, 26 miles away. A great excitement rippled through the crowd when the runners were seen in the distance at the far end of the Ram Das Puri field, car-rying the flame high as they ran up to the stage. The historic church in Chimayo is one of three homes of the torch in the United States, another the United Nations in New York, and the third the gravesite of President John F. Kennedy in Arlington, Virginia.

KWTC in the summer of 1987 was five weeks long, and a record number of wom-en from all over the world came to spend the summer in Española. Many had taken for granted the privilege of attending Khalsa Women's Training Camp. But now in the after-math of his infirmity, each day with the Siri Singh Sahib became even more precious.

"My intention is to let us show the world that the American woman is not a chick," the Siri Singh Sahib told them that summer. "She is an eagle, the symbol of a nation. I want to see you spread your wings with that power. That's what I want to see."[5]

And what a joyous summer it was! Against doctor's orders the Siri Singh Sahib lectured daily under the gold and white, big-top tent set in the cottonwood grove of the Gold House. In addition, Master Darshan Singh and his jatha, Nirmal Singh and Santokh Singh, taught daily kirtan classes. Baba Nihal Singh recited Rehiras in different homes in the sangat and langar was served every night, lending an atmosphere of cel-ebration to the day. Bhai Jiwan Singh sang daily in gurdwara, and the beat of WAHE GURU could be heard from the camp loudspeakers all over the Sombrillo valley.

Now in its 11th year, KWTC had taken on a nature and spirit of its own. "Sending my wife to KWTC is like sending myself to sadhana each morning—it's a conscious decision I never regret. She spends day after day with her spiritual teacher, she is with ladies like herself, and she can learn many new things. The ways in which a woman is powerful are myriad: she can channel her energy through yoga; she can solidify her connection with her Guru through kirtan; she can express her ability and grace as a woman through contact with her sisters; and she can refine her devotion to service through karma yoga. She is both a teacher and a student."[6]

The Furmaan Khalsa

In the spring of 1983 the Siri Singh Sahib wrote 108 remarkable poems over a three-week period. During that incredibly short time, no matter where he was or what he was doing, it was as if a voice was speaking to him and he would stop and dictate a complete poem in the meter and rhythm of Gurbani. If he was teaching White Tantric Yoga, he dictated the poem where he sat, to whomever was capable of writing Gurmukhi script. This inspired work of art emerged as an extraordinary collection of poems, written by various hands and pens on whatever scrap of paper was available at the time.

After several people attempted to translate these poems, the Siri Singh Sahib gave the job to Singh Sahib Guruka Singh Khalsa. As a blessing and a labor of love, he completed the job and published these poems in 1987 under the title *Furmaan Khalsa*.

"When people see the throne of Guru Ram Das rise in glory through time and space as the Dharma evolves, they are going to see this as the seminal volume that captured the essence of what the throne of Guru Ram Das is, the throne of Raj Yog, and those who live their lives in dedication to the throne of Raj Yog. It is the single thing written that the Siri Singh Sahib will be most remembered for, because although we have a lot of lectures that are transcribed, these are poems that he has composed directly himself."[7]

This amazing work had a far-reaching significance, written, in fact, for the future generations of Khalsa. As described by the Siri Singh Sahib, "If all my lectures and writings were lost, and nothing remained of my teachings, everything is told in this book. Just by studying this one book, you can understand the essence of all my teachings."

Hail! Hail Guru Ram Das and Heal the World!

The power of healing became a central focus for the sangat and the object of their prayers and meditation. The Golden Temple needed healing; the Siri Singh Sahib needed healing; the psyche of the Sikh Nation needed healing. The sangat called on that upon which they had relied for the past 20 years, the hand of Guru Ram Das through the power of prayer.

"Guru Ram Das is a very, very active Guru. He works miracles, just let Him work.

Just do it in His name. Say 'Hail Guru Ram Das and Heal the World,' and you shall never need me. You shall need nothing! Just hail and heal. Hail Guru Ram Das and heal in His Name. There is a job to be done, my friends, and the truth is by camouflage and manipulation it cannot be done. It takes a pure heart and a very simple approach.

"If you want to see Guru Ram Das, 'Hail!' and He shall heal you and heal your surroundings. Make Him personal; don't put Him outside. Don't make a statue out of Him in the sense that He is outside yourself. See Him in you. There is only one line that you can live with: *Ang Sang Wahe Guru.* 'The life and limb, the fiber of my being, belongs to Wahe Guru.' Make Him your personal Guru. Very personal."[8]

"Now is the time to heal the world at large by hailing Guru Ram Das. Let Guru work. Let Guru come through. Guru is *samarath* (powerful). Guru is *partakh* (manifest). Guru is perfect. Guru is competent. Guru is infinite. Guru is our ultimate anchor. So, hail Guru Ram Das and heal in His name. You don't have to be afraid. If you want to work miracles, just let Him work. Hail Guru Ram Das and heal the world in His Name! You shall need nothing else."[9]

The Power of Prayer

With the sixth of the month gurdwara program for the Akal Takhat continuing, and meditations being conducted for the Siri Singh Sahib's health, the faith of the sangat rested on the manifested power of prayer.

"You must understand that you are an individual magnetic psyche working in a huge magnetic field. This pranic energy by which we live is nothing but an electromagnetic field. This whole universe is the coexistence of a working electromagnetic field. Each individual magnetic field has its own frequency, its own rhythm, its own axis, and its own orbit. You are in perfect harmony with another person whenever you cross the range of another field and the psyches intertwine. And for your prayers to be effective, your frequency must intertwine with the infinite electromagnetic field, the Creator.

"For any progressive contribution you make, you must have the absolute connection with the entire psyche of the electromagnetic computerized system, which we call 'God.' You project at a certain frequency through your little tiny electromagnetic field to the universal psyche. If your signals are correct the results shall be perfect. Your signals are called prayers. The creatures send prayers to the Creator. The Guru says:

Savaa laakh se ek laraanoo
Gobind Singh naan kahaaoo

If a hundred twenty-five thousand come to fight me,
I will win over them.

Guru Gobind Singh

Chapter Five

"That only means that one electromagnetic psyche is so perfect and computerized that it can send a signal to the master electromagnetic psyche to rearrange the strength and coordinate the fulfillment by that psyche that shall give the victory.

"So don't misunderstand that prayer is only that which you say or utter. Prayer is also that, but real prayer means attention. Where you, your soul, your mind pay attention, that is called prayer. Physically, when we fold our hands, close our eyes, and worship, that is only getting the scene together."[10]

"Prayer is not talking to God. Communicating with your soul is not necessary. The soul is already there, communicating even without your help. Prayer is tapping energy from your own unknown. And the only channel through which your own unknown can reach you for help is the power of your own prayer. When the known and the unknown are united in the oneness of the self, God is alive.

"Therefore the power of prayer has to be continuous. Those who see whatever is around them as God are always tapped into their known and unknown. One who sees that realm of consciousness, feels it, and experiences it is called a living prayer. God is so great that whosoever touches that greatness must appreciate it. And the appreciation of God is prayer.

"Prayer goes where it will. And when the heart gets into the prayer, every beat of the heart creates a miracle. Man's power is in his prayer. And where prayer goes, God follows. That is one area where Almighty God follows man. That is the power of prayer."[11]

The Healers of Sikh Dharma
Because of the expansive nature of the meditative mind, people in the sangat developed a natural inclination to be healers. All over the world Sikhs were appearing as doctors, chiropractors, acupuncturists, and counselors. As a natural evolution from the self-healing practice of Kundalini Yoga, the students of 3HO were making their mark in the world of alternative healing. The Siri Singh Sahib taught his students to approach healing in a holistic manner—body, mind, and spirit, through the "Science of Humanology."

"The art of healing, the art of ecstasy, the art of God-consciousness has millions of names in mystic terms. It has to do with rhythm and reality. When the body is in rhythm, there is ease. When the body or any part of the body goes out of rhythm, there is disease. Disease is nothing but an out-of-rhythm body. When the mind is out of rhythm, there is neither a body nor a soul, because without the mind there is no reality. There can be no happiness."[12]

In December of 1979 during a teaching tour in Alaska, the Siri Singh Sahib dictated the first of a series of herbal formulas based on Ayurveda, the original great healing system of India. Unlike drugs, which are synthesized chemicals used to manipulate body processes, herbs are natural, unprocessed substances with specific properties that help the body to harmonize and increase organ and glandular functioning to appropriate levels. "**Doctors prescribe. Medicines cure. Herbs heal.**"

Healthcare practitioners find that patients respond well to yogic techniques. It reaches a part of their psyche that other, more traditional forms of medicine cannot treat. As Singh Sahib Dr. Gurusahay Singh Khalsa, a chiropractic doctor from Atlanta, Georgia, explains, "I spend as much time helping people to reduce their stress and just enjoy life as I do working on relieving physical pain. I often give them meditation techniques as part of the healing process. I would never have learned from traditional medicine or even alternative medicine the things I have learned from the 3HO teachings."

In order to share the growing knowledge base generated from the Siri Singh Sahib's teachings, in 1982 the Khalsa Chiropractic Association was formed. They realized that they could help each other to spread the teachings and focus the unique healing capabilities of these teachings through their practice as Doctors of Chiropractic. Now this group has over 20 chiropractors who all share the name "Dr. Khalsa." They meet yearly for one week to talk about what they have learned, how they incorporate these things into their practice, and also to work to heal each other so that they can better heal their patients.

Many Sikh doctors, nurses, and counselors serve in the field of AIDS care, offering their positivity and vitality to those who are facing this traumatic and destructive disease. Through yoga and meditation, their patients are given a life-affirming experience, reconnecting them to their own source of internal healing—their life force. People don't heal in isolation, and through yoga and meditation the patient finds a direct way to connect to the psyche of the planet.

Sardarni Sahiba Dr. Shanti Shanti Kaur Khalsa, a medical family therapist in Los Angeles, works with AIDS patients and other people facing life-threatening medical conditions. "Yoga actually has a biological basis for helping people get well," she states. "It works on the glandular system, the nervous system, the lymphatic system. It supports your immune system and through the breathing techniques, it breaks old emotional responses and physiological patterns. Yoga can be a useful tool for health recovery."

A Portrait of Strength and Grace
Bibiji Inderjit Kaur, the Siri Singh Sahib's wife, serves the Panth Khalsa in many ways: teaching, counseling, inspiring, and uplifting the Sikhs all over the world. Throughout the years, her classes and workshops in marriage and child-raising at Solstice and KWTC have helped shape a new generation of Khalsa.

After arriving and relocating her family in America, she returned to school and earned her masters degree and then her PhD in psychology in 1989. From there she went on to obtain her state license to practice as a clinical therapist. Bibiji is recognized by her associates as a spiritual leader and talented counselor. She serves on numerous boards including three consecutive terms as a member of the Governor's Youth Authority Advisory Board in New Mexico. This board helps create and develop improved social and educational opportunities for the youth. In 1993 she was named by Governor Bruce King as one of the founding members of the New Mexico Counseling and Therapists Practice Board.

One of her most significant projects has been her recent work with the United Nations. The 3HO Foundation was accepted as a Non-Governmental Organization Member of the United Nations in 1994. Representing 3HO, Bibiji led a delegation of western Sikhs to the United Nations International Conference on Population and Development in Cairo, Egypt, in September, 1994. This historical conference laid a foundation of cooperation among nations and diverse cultural groups for dealing with the serious problem of overpopulation in the world today. She held the crowd in rapt attention as she spoke on the plight of youth in crisis around the world, and the members of the Sikh delegation were flooded with questions about Sikh Dharma. As a result Kundalini Yoga classes were established in Cairo under the guidance of Sardarni Sahiba Tarn Taran Kaur Khalsa of 3HO Europe.

In 1985 Bibiji was appointed Bhai Sahiba of the Khalsa Council, the Chief Minister for Sikh Dharma of the Western Hemisphere. Her role on the Khalsa Council is to uphold the integrity of the Sikh Rehit Maryada in all of the Council's proceedings. The Bhai Sahiba's section has produced several books and publications in English to instruct people in the Sikh teachings. Some of these projects include *Gurdwara Protocol,* the *Amrit Ceremony,* the *Anand Karaj* (Sikh wedding ceremony) and the *Sikh Rehit Maryada.* Many of these books have been translated into foreign languages to serve the sangats in Mexico, Europe, and Asia.

Manner, Mission and Magnitude

In 1985 the Siri Singh Sahib expanded the structure of the Khalsa Council, and it grew in size from two dozen to over 100 members. Mukhia Sardarni Sahiba Sardarni Guru Amrit Kaur Khalsa was appointed as the Secretary General to oversee and guide the operations of the Council. As the sangat strove to shoulder more of the responsibility for Sikh Dharma of the Western Hemisphere, the role and purpose of the Khalsa Council expanded.

The Khalsa Council structure, which serves in this form today, is made up of five main sections:

The Head Table is staffed by the Chancellor of Sikh Dharma, the Chief Whip, the Principle Recorder, and an elected Chairman of the Khalsa Council whose term rotates every two years.

The Government Section is headed by the Secretary General and consists of the Secretariat staff, an Assistant Chancellor who serves as Parliamentarian, and all Regional administrative personnel. The Executive Secretary sits in the Government Section as well and holds veto power on all motions of the Council, ensuring that the long-term stability of Sikh Dharma is safeguarded.

The House is made up of 52 members, filled by ministers from around the world.

Their main function is to represent the needs of the sangat to the Khalsa Council, and to communicate with the sangats of their area on the work and progress of the Council. A Speaker of the House is elected every two years and acts as their leader and spokesman.

The Bhai Sahiba's Section is an 11-member group that oversees that the values and protocol of Sikh Dharma are maintained. This section is responsible for all religious ceremonies and protocol during the meetings, including opening the Khalsa Council session with Japaji Sahib, and the daily interpretation of the Hukam.

The Council of Nominees is made up of 11 members who represent the eyes and ears of the Siri Singh Sahib. They sit in silence, but as a group hold veto power over all of the Khalsa Council motions. They report directly to the Siri Singh Sahib as a grassroots view of the actions of the Council.

Since 1985 the following sections were added to the Khalsa Council:

Members in Training are a group of not more than 11 members who sit in the House Section. This section can participate in Council discussions but cannot vote on motions. In all other sections Khalsa Council members are selected and appointed by the Siri Singh Sahib. However, Members in Training may petition a seat from Siri Singh Sahib after gathering 52 signatures from the community they wish to represent.

The Youth Section is a five-member section created to give a voice to the youth of the Khalsa Nation. They may participate in all debate and discussion, but do not hold the privilege of voting. Additional seats are reserved for the Sikh Youth Federation of Canada to encourage and facilitate their involvement in the administration of Sikh Dharma and to express their ideas as a means of fulfilling their vision for the future.

In 1986, **the European Khalsa Council** was formed based on the model of the Khalsa Council. This body deals with the annual European Yoga Festival, the expansion of Sikh Dharma in Europe, and other topics unique to the European sangat.

In April of 1990, the Khalsa Council mapped out the programs and agendas of primary concern for the remainder of this decade. The priorities they established were: Children of the Khalsa, Prosperity, Living and Spreading the Teachings, and Leadership.

In 1991, the Khalsa Council created a Board of Trustees with Mukhia Singh Sahib Daya Singh Khalsa as chairman to deal with the many pressing issues relating to Sikh youth. The Board of Trustees formed the Office of Youth Affairs to administer the various youth programs and respond to the needs of the Khalsa children. Sardarni Sahiba Kirn Kaur Khalsa was appointed as the pioneer Executive Director of the Office of Youth Affairs. This office is responsible for the Khalsa Youth Camps, the Sikh Dharma Foreign Education Program, and other projects set up for the youth of the Khalsa.

As the health of the Siri Singh Sahib became more precarious, the weight of the leadership of Sikh Dharma came to rest on the shoulders of the Secretariat and the Khalsa Council. In December of 1990 the Siri Singh Sahib addressed the Khalsa Council:

"Every man and woman must have manners, mission, and magnitude. These are aspects of life that you cannot change. In us there is a capacity. It is not a factor of how we eat, sleep, think, or how much money we have. It is in our manners. If those manner are spiritual, we are spiritual, and our mission is spiritually based. The magnitude of life can be infinity, and it is achievable. There is only one positive way to live: those who live in yesterday are miserable, those who live today are depressed, those who welcome tomorrow are prosperous and hopeful. It is the attitude of magnitude and the manners of the mission that makes the man!"[13]

The bylaws of the Khalsa Council lay out the details of the organization of the Khalsa Council. This document clearly delineates how the next Siri Singh Sahib will be chosen and how he or she will fill the post. Still, many people were fraught with insecurity at the thought of who could possibly fill the shoes of Yogi Bhajan when that time came.

"A question that is asked is: 'Siri Singh Sahib, what will happen after you? Yogiji, what do you think will happen?'

"I'll tell you what I think, and I would like to explain that to you today. Sikh Dharma belongs to the father of this Dharma, Guru Gobind Singh. First He was Gobind Rai, then He was exalted to Guru Gobind Singh. That is a miracle! That is a '*karamat!*' That person as a personified god could create four sons, Baba Ajeet Singh, Baba Jujhar Singh, Baba Zorawar Singh, and Baba Fateh Singh who could face life and marry the bride we call death. Such fearlessness. No vengeance. The beauty of duty was examined, exalted, done, and completed. So please understand, whatever is happening is by Guru's Will. The father, the leader, the owner, and the guide is Guru Gobind Singh. The Guru is *Siri Guru Granth Sahib* and the body is the Khalsa. This system is set by the Guru and this system shall be followed by the Khalsa. Have no fear because I have no fear. Have no reservations because I have no reservations. The tide is in now, and the sea is open to us!"[14]

In the fall of 1991, the Siri Singh Sahib authored the "Constitution of the Administrative Council of Every Sadh Sangat." This document is a working blueprint for the format of sangat management. It establishes a Khalsa Administrative Council in each sangat, designed to represent the people by dividing the body of the sangat into four constituencies named for each of the sons of Guru Gobind Singh. Each constituency elects one or more representatives who sit on the council, voicing the needs and opinions of the people they serve. Completing the Khalsa Administrative Council is an appointed Senate body, the Ashram Director, and an Executive Secretary. "On that style and pattern, the community will grow democratically serving every facet and figuring out our future."[15]

The Secretariat of Sikh Dharma International Headquarters

The Secretariat of Sikh Dharma has taken a huge responsibility in serving the Sikhs of the Western Hemisphere. Staffed by many dedicated individuals devoted to the mission of Guru Ram Das, the Secretariat is the hub of Sikh Dharma, 3HO Foundation, and the

Office of the Siri Singh Sahib. From the Secretariat come the many publications, camps, Gurpurb celebrations, and classes hosted by Sikh Dharma and 3HO. They host visitors and guests from all nations and walks of life. They are responsible for raising funds and managing the assets of Sikh Dharma, ensuring a rich heritage for the children of the Khalsa and the generations to follow. They provide guidance and counsel to the thousands of people who write and call with questions and problems.

Under the leadership of Mukhia Sardarni Sahiba Sardarni Guru Amrit Kaur Khalsa, the Office of the Secretary General directs and guides the departments and offices of the Sikh Dharma Secretariat. Her vision and long-term planning focus their efforts and direction.

Mukhia Sardarni Sahiba Shakti Parwha Kaur Khalsa has upheld and maintained the Office of the Executive Secretary since the very beginning of Sikh Dharma in the West, when the Secretariat was just an idea in the mind of the Siri Singh Sahib. She has stood as the guardian of the ideals and values, the assets and properties of Sikh Dharma for 25 years, making sure that all systems operate within the established order. Her wisdom and counsel have been sought by hundreds of people spanning three generations. Her newsletter, *The Science of Keeping Up!,* is the longest standing publication of the Secretariat. It keeps the sangat informed of trends and current events in all the faraway places of the world where 3HO Foundation flourishes. This journal includes the latest Kundalini Yoga information and teachings given by Yogi Bhajan on all aspects of life. Today, she still teaches the beginning Kundalini Yoga course in Los Angeles that was originally started 25 years ago by Yogi Bhajan.

The Office of the Siri Singh Sahib continually buzzes with energy and activity. Mukhia Sardarni Sahiba Nirinjan Kaur Khalsa, Chief of Staff, directs and manages the flow of activity in and around the Siri Singh Sahib, managing his busy appointment and touring schedule. Under his direction she administers the Secretariat in New Mexico, which includes the Office of Youth Affairs, the Fund Development Office, the Office of the Teachings, the Events Office, and the Public Affairs Office. Sardarni Sahiba Siri Simran Kaur Khalsa is the personal secretary of the Siri Singh Sahib, fielding the thousands of letters and inquiries that come to him each year.

In 1969 Sardarni Sahiba Soorya Kaur Khalsa was the first woman to take Sikh vows, and with her pioneering spirit she ventured forth and opened many ashrams across the country. Her role as a staff member in the Sikh Dharma Secretariat has included many special projects, including 3HO SuperHealth, *Beads of Truth,* and the Sikh Dharma Archives, documenting the growth of Sikh Dharma in pictures with her photographic skills.

Sardarni Sahiba Sopurkh Kaur Khalsa is the Comptroller General of the Sikh Dharma Secretariat and the President of Khalsa International Trading. Responsible for all the financial matters of Sikh Dharma of the Western Hemisphere, she bears this heavy weight with dignity and grace. She is a woman of rare insight and vision, planning the economic stability of Sikh Dharma far into the future. Also serving the Financial Department of the Secretariat are Sardarni Sahiba Hari Simran Kaur Khalsa and many other devoted sevadars. Sardarni Sahiba Sat Simran Kaur Khalsa, Secretary of State, and Gobind Kaur Khalsa, the Assistant Secretary of State, oversee the management and development of the properties and vehicles owned by Sikh Dharma.

The Siri Singh Sahib plays an active role in businesses owned by Sikh Dharma. He keeps abreast of all business activity through his Chief Business Reviewer, Sardarni Sahiba Peraim Kaur Khalsa; Executive Secretary, Sardarni Sahiba Siri Karm Kaur Khalsa; Chief Business Secretary, Sardarni Sahiba Siri Ram Kaur Khalsa, and the Assistant Chief Business Secretary, Sumpuran Kaur Khalsa.

Since the 3HO Foundation was formed in 1969, the Secretariat has published a magazine entitled *Beads of Truth,* which chronicles the growth and progress of the organization. In the early days of 3HO, *Beads* was a critical information link to the hundreds of new ashrams that were formed. Filled with Sikh technology, Kundalini Yoga sets, vegetarian cooking recipes, and news of the sangat, *Beads of Truth* circulated around the world. Now that magazine has evolved into a sophisticated periodical of Sikh Dharma International and 3HO Foundation, publishing news and events as well as information on the technology of the new age.

In 1987, "Sikhnet" was created at the request of the Siri Singh Sahib. This computer bulletin board system broadcasts the news of the Secretariat and the Khalsa Council to the sangat, transcriptions of the Siri Singh Sahib's lectures, news from India, and selected wire service stories. At its peak, it had over 100 subscribers. By the end of 1994, Sikhnet evolved into a vast electronic mail system, linking the personal and business computers of Sikhs all over the United States and Canada.

The Children of the Dharma

Through the devastating years of the late 80s in the Punjab when the life of every Sikh was challenged and changed, the children of Sikh Dharma Foreign Education remained in school in India. This great act of faith by the parents of Sikh Dharma sent a clear message to the Panth in India that they were with them in prayer and in brotherhood. In 1986 Sardarni Sahiba Hari Kaur Khalsa and Singh Sahib Siri Akal Singh Khalsa joined the staff of SDFE in India.

With the environment still too dangerous for Sikhs to travel around India, the children came home for their winter breaks in 1987 and 1988. Baba Nihal Singh, Bhai Jiwan Singh, and Sardar Paramjeet Singh from Malaysia came to New Mexico and spent hours with the children teaching them Gurbani Kirtan and Sikh Rehit. Baba Nihal Singh used a timpani drum from a nearby elementary school to teach the children the rhythm of the large *Ranjit Nagara*. This giant drum was used during the days of Guru Gobind Singh in Anandpur Sahib. Today it is used to herald the arrival and departure of the *Siri Guru Granth Sahib* during gurdwara and to give dramatic emphasis to the Ardas.

Within a few years the SDFE program relocated down the mountain from Mussoorie to the Guru Ram Das Academy in Dehra Dun. Because the weather was more moderate in the lower altitude of Dehra Dun, the children were able to take their long break in the summer, allowing them to participate in the summer activities in Española.

Responding to the special needs of Khalsa teenagers, in 1988 the Siri Singh Sahib conceived a summer camp for the youth to challenge them and strengthen their spirits. The first "Survival Camp" was held in the mountains of Ram Das Puri in August. Today Survival Camp is a nonstop action packed adventure guaranteed to challenge and uplift the Khalsa youth. With a motto of "tough enough," activities include rock climbing, hiking, shooting, and martial arts.

During the winter break of 1989-1990, the school children were able to return to the Punjab for the first time since 1984 as the region struggled to regain normality. They camped at a farm near Anandpur Sahib and again were happily absorbed into life in rural India. Because the situation in Punjab was still very tense, they did not travel around to the villages as they had in past years, but were content to live in the simple harmony of green fields, water buffaloes, and spiritual practice.

It was unbearable for them to be in the Punjab and not visit the Harimandir Sahib. They were so close and yet the obstacles to traveling to Amritsar were enormous. However, one day in January, 1990, some of the camp leaders, Hari Kaur, Gurupreet Singh, and Fateh Singh could resist no longer, and went quietly into the city of Amritsar. As soon as they entered the Amritsar district they were followed by the military police who intimidated them with their unrelenting presence. In order to enter the Golden Temple complex they had to pass through a military checkpoint. They were searched thoroughly, as was every devotee who came to pray at the Golden Temple.

What they saw was more shocking than the sum of all the rumors and reports they had heard. Even after six years, many buildings were still blackened and gutted, reminders of the horrible battle that had occurred. Guru Nanak Nivas had two huge mortar holes in the side of the building, and the ancient markets that abutted the walls of the Golden Temple complex for hundreds of years were demolished, leaving a wide swath of cleared land. The beautiful and artful marble parkarma around the sarovar was ruined, crushed, and riddled with thousands of cracks made from the tracks of the heavy military tanks that had rolled onto the marble during the attack on the Akal Takhat. The Akal Takhat itself was a skeleton, with only the very first stages of re-building evident. The shadow of death hung in the air and it was as if screams of agony could still be heard if you listened carefully. When Gurupreet Singh knelt on the parkarma to bow, tears of grief and pain streamed down his face.

But still, it was the magnificent Harimandir Sahib. The beautiful Gurbani Kirtan echoed across the waters into the souls of the American Sikhs. There was an unusual profusion of sparrows that had come to roost in the Baba Buddha tree, chirping and twirping, creating a huge noise and flutter. Later the Siri Singh Sahib said, "These sparrows must be carrying the souls of the thousands of people who died here, not yet wanting to leave."

They were in the Golden Temple for a very short time before they prudently made their departure. On their way out a Nihung sitting on the parkarma looked up as they walked by and exclaimed loudly in English, "Oh look! It's the American Singhs! They've returned!"

Gurdwaras are Built on Western Soil

As the maturity and prosperity of the sangat increased, gurdwaras were raised in the sangats of the Western Hemisphere. The first gurdwara was built at the Siri Singh Sahib's ranch in Española, New Mexico in 1981. It was lovingly adorned with marble floors, beautiful stained glass and paintings of the ten Sikh Gurus. A giant steel kandha was mounted on the wall, dominating the room.

On Guru Gaddhee Day, 1984, the Guru Ram Das Ashram in Millis, Massachusetts, opened the doors of their newly built gurdwara. "There is no way to bespeak its value, to measure its worth, to delimit its preciousness, to explain the usefulness and beauty of this facet of our communal existence. It is the foundation stone of our life together. It is the linchpin of our lives. The very walls hymn the Creator!"[16]

In 1985, marble was installed on the floor of Guru Ram Das Ashram in Los Angeles. Beautifully carved doors and precious etched glass windows transformed the sadhana room into an exquisite gurdwara. "So although we are in deep sorrow that we cannot visit the House of Guru Ram Das in Amritsar now, we can close our eyes and transport ourselves into that same ecstasy of consciousness by cleaning the marble floor of Guru Ram Das Ashram."[17]

In the fall of 1989, plans were made in Española to expand the main ashram building into a gurdwara. Years ago the sangat had become too large to hold gurdwara services in the original building and had utilized a temporary building for that purpose. When Mukhia Singh Sahib Dr. Guruchander Singh Khalsa brought the idea of building a gurdwara to the Siri Singh Sahib, he said, "OK, I give you my blessing to do this. But I want to see the plans within seven days!" The plans were hastily produced but the Siri Singh Sahib was not totally satisfied. He told them they had to crown the building with a gold dome. No one had the money or the expertise to produce such a dome, so the Siri Singh Sahib was told it was impossible.

Construction on the gurdwara began immediately. All the work was done by people in the sangat as seva and funds for materials were donated from all over the world. The building rose from the ground with tall walls and a giant beamed ceiling in the style of New Mexico architecture. One day in October at 2:00 AM, they broke through the adjoining wall, opening the old sadhana room that contained the mural painted by Edward O'Brien into the grand hall of the new gurdwara.

Again and again the Siri Singh Sahib insisted that a gold dome must be built, and again he was told it was impossible. The fourth time he asked for it, Singh Sahib Simran Singh Khalsa came up with a design, and it was decided that it was indeed possible. The dome was built and covered with gold. Today, the gold dome shining in the sunlight can be seen from every desert hilltop in the area, as if calling the Sikhs of the Guru to prayer.

When the gurdwara was opened in July, 1990, the Siri Singh Sahib named it "Siri Takhat Sahib Takhat a Khalsa." He made the sangat understand that its purpose was bigger than just a local gurdwara. They had built something historical that had dramatically changed their lives, manifesting the Guru's will.

The Ancient Healing Walk of the Hopi's
In early 1990, the Siri Singh Sahib told his students a remarkable story. "When we first bought Guru Ram Das Puri, the sacred Elders of the Hopi Indians came to me to tell me about this land. The Hopis are the keepers of the ancient wisdom and history of the People. The Indians used to live up here, and down below where the valley is, in the town of Española, there was a huge lake. You can still go there and find old fish stuck in stone, and you don't know where it could come from in this desert. But that is what it was.

"Ram Das Puri was a common ground where the elders and warriors from all the different tribes used to gather once every hundred years to pray to the One Creator, the Great Spirit. But then there was a dry age of forty-two years. For forty-two years, not a drop of rain fell on this planet. Not one. And that huge lake dried up. The Indians had to move, and they went south into Mexico.

"That Hopi Indian said that Ram Das Puri was their ancient land, and that here they used to have a healing practice. So I said, 'How did you used to heal?' And this very old man said, 'Can we talk differently?' So we went by ourselves to the side, and he told me I should build a mile and a quarter circle like a Kundalini energy. I was shocked when I heard what he said, this man who was so old he couldn't see, couldn't walk, couldn't even get up by himself. He told me that anyone who will walk on his heels through that circle will be healed, it doesn't matter if he knows anything or not.

"He said, 'The Sacred Warriors must return here and meet in prayer. Purity and piety are the soul of the river that flows under this land. The sacred river of my Fathers and Grandfathers under our feet is our soul. If you want to be healed, walk the four directions in a circle, three and one-half times. Now the eagle is freed. The secret of the land has been told.'"

As part of Peace Prayer Day, 1990, a spiral track was cleared in the large field at Ram Das Puri, and the first healing walk was performed. The soft dirt on the track was carefully raked and groomed so that the participants of Peace Prayer Day could walk barefoot on their heels to the beat of the Native American drum. With solemnity, the Sacred Healing Walk took its place among the annual traditions of 3HO Foundation.

The Dawning of the Age of Aquarius
November 11, 1991, did not dawn as an ordinary day. The sun rose in the East as it has for millions of years and the humans awoke to another day on planet earth. But a

remarkable thing was occurring in the heavens. This day marked the beginning of the cusp of the Aquarian Age.

"Today, after two thousand years, Mars and Jupiter have crossed over and under. The change of the age has been established and now we are entering a seven-year period in which we will go through the cusp of the transmigration of one age into an other. Then the Age of Aquarius will start.

"In the Age of Aquarius, people will have a different language and people will have a different understanding. The process, projection, and perpetual preparedness of man shall be based on his subtle message. Man shall talk to the heavens and the heavens shall talk back to the earth at the same time. It won't be difficult for you. Just as a fax machine does it today, tomorrow you will not need that machine. You have your own thirty trillion mega-wattage in your brain and you will be in a posi- tion to read and transmit to other people whenever you feel like it. It has started already. Look! Today you are totally illiterate before your own children. Your own born kids can solve certain puzzles and run certain computers that you can't even think about doing.

"Rejoice! The Age of Aquarius has set in. The rulership of the Lord of this age is the *Siri Guru Granth Sahib.* Siri Guru Granth is the Guru of the Aquarian Age because it teaches subtly. When your subtlety is intact, your satellite is on the orbit, and mes- sages can go back and forth between you and God. Subtlety gives us crystal-clear clar- ity, not the opaqueness of subexistence. Humans cannot live anymore in subhuman consciousness. No candle wants to just smoke. It wants to be lit! That is what the Age of Aquarius is. That's what Sikh Dharma is all about. And that is our tomorrow."[18]

"In this Age of Aquarius, the human mind is an exalted mind. The Piscean Age was, 'I want to know, I want to search, I want to see.' And the Age of Aquarius is, 'It is known to me. I have no duality. I am the Power. I am Divine. I am Reality. I Am.'

"With this 'I Am,' there is a grace, there is a love, there is affection. Vastness. Not limited. Not shallowness. Whenever a person gives his or her personal self to him*self*, the person has achieved bliss. How beautiful it can be if you can realize that you are *realized.* Not that somebody else has to define you as realized. You realize that you are *realized.*"[19]

Sikh Dharma and the Red Bear

There are few colder places on the planet earth than Moscow in January. The air is so cold that if you breathe it directly you risk freezing the tissue in your lungs. But it was in January of 1990 that the Siri Singh Sahib and his staff traveled to Moscow in what was still the Soviet Union, for the Global Forum on the Environment. There were many delegates there from all over the world including the future Vice President of the United States, Al Gore. The meetings were informative and served to create a base of understanding be- tween nations as to the environmental problems facing the countries of the world.

During one evening event, the President of the Soviet Union, Mikhail Gorbachev,

The Quantum Impact of the Shabad Guru

We are entering a new period in the evolution of human consciousness that is characterized both by a rapid sense of change and, paradoxically, by the simultaneous awareness of certain constant truths. This difficult and tumultuous period in our history requires the mastery of specific technologies and tools in order for us to survive. The Shabad Guru is one of these unique tools. In fact, our usage and mastery of the Shabad Guru will have a quantum impact on our awareness and on our lives.

During this latter part of the twentieth century, the forefront of scientific research has been theoretical physics. Theoretical physics consists of the postulation and subsequent proof of the actual manner in which the universe is constructed. It is now understood that the composition of matter, that at first was believed to be comprised of minute particles called protons, neutrons, and electrons and later understood to consist of even smaller component particles is in fact simply energy; energy that is constantly transforming itself into different frequencies of vibration. Matter, science is discovering, is nothing more than a constant flow of changing ripples and waves in one cosmic sea of energy. When we understand that matter itself is, in reality, the interplay and patterns of energy waves, and that waves of energy are what we recognize as sound, it requires no great leap of faith to see that all form in nature is manifested and constantly affected by causative sound.

There are patterns in the structure and rhythm of Gurbani that are templates of infinity. The technology of Shabad Guru is that this sound current, this wave of energy, was created by a human being who had entered into the state of ecstasy, the completely neutral mind. In this neutral mind, he had the true experience of life and expressed it in the form and science of Gurbani. We can re-create this experience of infinity through the recitation of Gurbani.

Gurbani gives you, embedded in the language, in the reflexology, and in the concepts, the experience of infinity by engaging the neutral mind, allowing you to act in a spontaneous flow. That's the concept. Shabad Guru gives us that internal point of reference so that we can handle everything that comes to us without being thrown off center. It gives the ability to integrate two perspectives, the subjective and the objective, because it provides the neutral reference point. When each part of ourselves is fully integrated, we become natural and spontaneous. We become Saibhang; self contained, self-integrated illumination. That is the quantum impact of the Shabad Guru.

Singh Sahib Guruka Singh Khalsa
March 30, 1995

173

was present to welcome and meet the delegates. From the far side of a large reception hall President Gorbachev caught sight of the Siri Singh Sahib in his distinctive white robe and turban, and cut a path through the crowd directly toward him. He came up to him with a big smile, grabbed his hand, and started pumping it while exclaiming, "You are the man on the tea box!"

As it turned out, the Sikhs had sent President Gorbachev a case of Yogi Tea a few years earlier. He was delighted with the spicy, sweet drink and remembered fondly the simple, unsolicited gift.

In a subsequent visit the Siri Singh Sahib established the 3HO Foundation in the Soviet Union. Teachers were trained and Kundalini Yoga classes quickly gained momentum. That summer 20 students took vows to live as Sikhs of the Guru, and turbans, karas, and kacheras were arranged for each of them.

Bibiji Inderjit Kaur went to Moscow in early May of 1991 to promote the 3HO Superhealth program in the Soviet Union. She traveled to Turkistan where a Superhealth Center was opened to treat the extensive problem of alcohol addiction that afflicts an estimated one-third of the population in Russia. She visited many cities and was graciously received at each stop.

After the dissolution of the Soviet Union, western Sikhs returned to Russia to teach regular classes and support the small local Sikh sangat. Business enterprises were explored and steps were taken for lasting contact with the Russian people.

The Strength of a Community United

When Sardarni Sahiba Guru Raj Kaur Khalsa moved to Vancouver, Canada in 1973 to open the Guru Ram Das Ashram, she was dismayed at the status of the Indian Sikh community. In Vancouver the Sikh population is substantial. Over 50,000 Sikhs live there, as they had been immigrating to that part of Canada since the turn of the century. They came from India in large numbers during the 60s and 70s to seek out a better life for themselves and their families. Very few Sikhs who came to the West kept the Rehit: long hair, turban, and beard. This marked them as foreigners, immigrants, a status and image that they wished to shed quickly. Those Sikhs who tried to keep their turban and beards often experienced oppressive discrimination, both socially and in the workplace. Although Canada has recently made great changes, in the early 70s if you were not white and Christian, you had a very hard time living in Canadian society. For many Indian immigrants, the first stop from the airport upon arriving in the West was the barber shop. The situation with the gurdwaras in Vancouver was indicative of the low point to which the Sikh community had sunk. During gurdwara programs head covers were worn by very few people, and the current topic of debate was whether or not to install pews in the gurdwara instead of sitting on the floor in the Sikh tradition.

When the Guru Ram Das Ashram was first opened, yoga classes were offered, and contact was made with the local Sikh community. Gurudeep Singh Atwal, a strong

Sikh who had maintained his Rehit, established close ties with the new Sikhs. They worked together to slowly strengthen and rebuild the Sikh identity in Vancouver. Guru Raj Kaur Khalsa began teaching "Sunday School" in the local gurdwara, and this was the first time some of the Indian children had heard the stories of the Sikh Gurus in a way they could understand.

The first priority was to involve the Sikh youth in the beauty and strength of their heritage. At the Siri Singh Sahib's direction, Guru Raj Kaur and Gurudeep Singh worked together to establish the Sikh Youth Federation of Canada, giving these Sikhs a forum to express their needs, ask questions, and seek their own fulfillment in the teachings of the Sikh Gurus. The Sikh Youth Federation grew into a mighty force, challenging the status quo. They offered moral support to those Sikhs who wanted to maintain their long hair and turban, and legal support in employment discrimination and civil rights cases. The Sikh Youth Federation founded a newsletter reaching out to the thousands of Sikhs in the area building up their community identity. They started bringing Ragi Jathas to Canada from India, filling the gurdwaras with beautiful and inspiring Gurbani Kirtan. Over the past 22 years, those same people have grown into the leaders of the vibrant and devoted Sikh community in Vancouver today.

Little by little, the community began to change and awaken to its proud identity as Sikhs. When the Golden Temple was attacked in 1984, an avalanche of Sikhs came back to their spiritual roots. Suddenly, it struck their hearts what it meant to be a Sikh, and together the east and west communities worked for a greater Sikh strength. Singh Sahib Swarn Singh Pattar was one such Sikh, reforming his life and rededicating himself as a Sikh after the tragedy of 1984. Today he serves the community as a minister of Sikh Dharma, participates in the Khalsa Council, and with his family, opens his home to the Sikhs of the Guru.

In Calgary, Sardarni Sahiba Dr. Harjot Kaur is an outstanding Gursikh woman, serving her community as a leader and teacher. She stands as a delegate of both the east and west Sikh communities and is known for her unshakable devotion. She is a valued member of the Khalsa Council and works closely with the Siri Singh Sahib.

In America also, a delicate weaving of communities has been occurring over the past 25 years. In Phoenix, Arizona, the Guru Nanak Gurdwara is a tribute to the mutual respect and cooperation between the Indian and American Sikh communities. The Indian traditions, attitude of service, and inborn devotion to the Guru's Word were deeply admired by the Americans who did not have the benefit of being raised in a Sikh family. And in turn the impassioned search for Truth and the revival of the Sikh technology by the American Sikhs served to inspire and rejuvenate the Indian community. Both cultures learned from each other and merged in a mutual and lasting respect. In the Guru Nanak Gurdwara, American and Indian ragis play Gurbani Kirtan together, Guru's Hukam is read in Gurmukhi, English, and Punjabi, and the children of both cultures attend classes and outings together. Originally established as a 3HO ashram, the Guru Nanak Gurdwara is now jointly managed, serving the Sikh community as a unified whole.

A Holy Man Among Diplomats

From the time the Siri Singh Sahib first arrived in the United States, he was keenly aware of local politics. He understood that a community such as the Sikhs, who are distinct in their appearance and customs, must work to serve and contribute to the society in which they live.

In his home state of New Mexico, the Siri Singh Sahib first met Governor Bruce King in 1970. Governor King went on to be the only three-time governor in the history of New Mexico, and the King family remained good friends of the Sikh Community throughout this time. As Governor King remembers: "I started in these parts as a County Commissioner, so I remember that this land used to be a windswept plain. When the Sikhs first settled here, I said, 'Well one windy day and they'll be gone.' So when you see all the beautiful green trees and plants they have established here, well then you realize the great asset that they have been, not only to this community but to the State of New Mexico!"[20]

The Sikh community in New Mexico became very involved in the political profile of the State. Mukhia Singh Sahib Daya Singh Khalsa, an active participant in state politics, explains it as follows: "We consider it an interest in public affairs rather than politics. One of the defining aspects of Sikh Dharma is that it is not a religion where you worship in one way and live your life in another way. It is a lifestyle, a unified way of life. What comes naturally out of that belief is that a Sikh needs to make a contribution not only to his own inner life or the small community around him but to the entire community as a whole."

Throughout the years, all types of politicians, both Democratic and Republican, visited the ranch to seek the advice and endorsement of the Siri Singh Sahib. In an election year it was considered a prudent course of action for any candidate to schedule a luncheon with the Siri Singh Sahib. He was renowned as a holy man among diplomats and a diplomat among holy men.

At his birthday party each year, the guest list reads like a Who's Who of state politics. A bipartisan gathering of senators, congressmen, governors, and all kinds of elected state officials join leaders from the religious community, family, and friends to celebrate the birthday of this well loved public figure.

"Yogi's birthday party is a must," US Representative Bill Richardson said affectionately. "That and Peace Prayer Day in the summer. It's smart not to miss those two occasions. [They] are players in the political scene in New Mexico."[21]

The political leaders of the state show genuine respect for the mission of Sikh Dharma. Attorney General Tom Udal expressed this during the Siri Singh Sahib's 1993 birthday party: "The thing about the community that [Yogi Bhajan] has started here, and has grown, and has become so much a part of Northern New Mexico, is that they are a wonderful model. In these times, many of the things that happen in our communities tend to divide us; divide us along economic lines and lines of race. [The Sikh Community], Yogiji, you should be very proud of. In terms of working with each other, sharing with each other, caring about each other, it serves as a model of the direction in which we ought to be heading."[22]

In 1993 the Sikhs participated in the inauguration of the President of the United States, Bill Clinton. The Siri Singh Sahib's white robes and turban stood out among the Democratic leaders who assembled for the swearing-in ceremonies. During the inaugural parade, President Clinton came up to the Sikhs to personally express his appreciation for their support.

Return to the Beloved Harimandir Sahib

After nine long years of prayer, the Siri Singh Sahib and a yatra of 160 people finally were able to return to the holy city of Amritsar in the spring of 1993. Traveling nonstop with very little sleep, on and off planes, buses, and trains they finally arrived with much anticipation at the gates of the Golden Temple complex. Purposely, the Siri Singh Sahib waited until the sun had set and the merciful cover of darkness had descended on the Harimandir Sahib so that the damage done in 1984 would not be so painfully visible. Still he was shocked as he made his rounds of the parkarma and saw the twisted skeletons of burned buses and cars and the smoke-blackened buildings that remained.

As the group made its way into the Harimandir Sahib, they were once again enchanted with the beauty and majesty of the House of Guru Ram Das. For some it was their first visit, for which they had prayed for years. Even though they had seen a hundred pictures and heard a thousand stories, they were unprepared for the magnificence of the Harimandir Sahib. Sarab Shakti Kaur, the young daughter of Mukhia Singh Sahib Hari Jiwan Singh Khalsa, Chief of Protocol to the Siri Singh Sahib, looked with wide-eyed amazement as she entered the Golden Temple for the first time. She said with a loud voice, "Oh God, look! It's all gold! We are rich!" People stopped in surprise to look at her, and the expression of ecstasy in that child's eyes brought smiles to their faces.

The group traveled throughout the Punjab and were welcomed with overwhelming hospitality and great joy everywhere they went. Throngs of people virtually mobbed the Siri Singh Sahib when he addressed the jubilant crowds at Jalandhar, Ludhiana, and Ambala. In this one week the hearts of the Indian people were reawakened to the goal of unity with their brothers and sisters from America. Seeing the western Khalsa on tour again symbolized to many that things were finally returning to normal in the Punjab.

"I think that Guru Ram Das was with us even more than we were with Him. With every step in India, '*Dhan dhan Raam Daas Gur, Jin siriaa tinai savaariaa. Pooree hoee karaamaat, aap sirjanhaarai dhaariaa.*' There was miracle after miracle! The eagerness and joy you brought to the Khalsa made the Khalsa open their hearts to you. It is my prayer that you will fulfill the prophecy, each one of you, as a representative. Let His will prevail now, and this planet will not be the same again. The whole Punjab woke up. The people had hope again."[23]

Santo, Ram Das Sarovar Neekaa

We get out of the cars at the Clock Tower Bazaar, and the gold light from the Harimandir Sahib can be seen shining through the Clock Tower arch. The Siri Singh Sahib moves with an anxious gait, urgent and expectant, and we shuffle to keep up with him. He is simply dressed, wrapped in two light shawls. He would have looked like a humble saint except that he wears his beautiful kirpan and carries his gold sword, giving him the appearance of a warrior king.

Walking through the arches of the Clock Tower and descending the steps onto the parkarma, the serenity of the Harimandir Sahib at Amrit Vela folds over you like a blanket. The air is cool and smells clean and humid. The light on the Golden Temple saturates the darkness with brilliant gold, and the reflection in the sarovar is dazzling. As he steps onto the parkarma with folded hands and his face turned to the Harimandir Sahib, the Siri Singh Sahib bows low and lays his forehead on the cool marble. He stays there for a long time, and the sound of Gurbani Kirtan echoes across the waters.

He rises, turns to the left and walks down the parkarma. Stopping at the Dukh Bhanjan Baree tree, he again turns to face the Harimandir Sahib with folded hands. He lays his hands on the trunk of the Dukh Bhanjan Baree and murmurs an unheard prayer, soft and lovingly. Taking off his shawls, he leaves them by the tree and in the chilly air he carefully walks down the marble steps to the water's edge.

A breeze picks up and the water in the sarovar ripples, causing the gold reflection from the Harimandir Sahib to sparkle off the water like so many gems and jewels. The kirtan has a distant, muted quality as it floats over the waters. He lifts his foot for the final step into the water, and there is a brief pause in the kirtan as the shabad changes. Then when his toe enters the water, the clear words of the shabad resounds: Santo, Raam Daas sarovar neekaa. Oh saints, come and bathe in the tank of Ram Das.

"Oh, Wha!" he said with tears streaming down his face, "Listen to the kirtan!"

The air, water, and ether had come together in perfect harmony to balance his fire, and the moment was crystallized in time. After nine long years, it was a beautiful welcome, an outstretching of open arms, from the home of his Guru.

The Siri Singh Sahib's political efforts were highlighted by a personal audience with the Prime Minister P.V. Narasimha Rao. The Prime Minister offered his commitment to working toward peace in the Punjab and gave his full assurance of his willingness to work with the Sikhs. He welcomed the western Khalsa and openly apologized for the suffering the community sustained by being prohibited from visiting the Golden Temple.

When in Amritsar the Khalsa women again requested the privilege to clean the floors of the Golden Temple during the Amrit Vela. With great hope and high spirits a group of Khalsa women gathered outside the gates at 11:30 PM with the other people waiting to do seva, but when the time came to enter the women were denied. "It never occurred to me that I would not be let in," said Siri Trang Kaur Khalsa. "I am Khalsa, and I serve my community and my Guru with the full responsibility of Khalsa. How could they, in their consciousness, lock us out?"

The situation became very tense, angry voices were heard, and extra guards were posted to make certain the ladies would not enter the Harimandir Sahib. Together they sat with a growing number of people gathering with them in support, chanting *Guru Guru Wahe Guru Guru Ram Das Guru* until the doors were opened to the public at 3:00 AM. Confirmed in the belief that it is a blessing as Khalsa to do seva at the Harimandir Sahib, the jatha left Amritsar with the sincere prayer that this brahministic and archaic rule would be rescinded.

"How can you let your temple be managed by those who do not even understand the meaning of the word 'Khalsa?' They have no eyes. They say, 'That is a woman and that is a man.' Can you believe this? It is shocking to me. Khalsa is Khalsa, and there is no man and no woman. To a certain extent man and woman do exist, but when one is a Khalsa, it is the purity, and the piety, and the ecstasy, and that part of the self which is not ours."[24]

Strength and Expansion in the 90s

During the 1893 World's Fair in Chicago, a forum known as the Parliament of the World's Religions convened. This was the first formal meeting in the history of the world where all of the major religions sat together in prayer and discussion. Nineteen ninety-three marked the centennial celebration of this great event, and the Parliament of the World's Religions met once again in a spirit of prayerful harmony. The Siri Singh Sahib participated in lectures and panel discussions, promoting dialog and cooperation among the different religious communities.

The camps and events of 3HO had grown significantly, proving to be the central cohesive factor among the 3HO family. Khalsa Women's Training Camp remained the center of summer activities and expanded to camps in Canada, Mexico, and Europe, reaching hundreds of women who couldn't travel to New Mexico.

In 1994, the 3HO International Kundalini Yoga Teachers Association was formed, celebrating the 25th anniversary of the 3HO Foundation. With over 600 people on the initial roster, the need for a consolidated teachers organization was evident. In June of 1994 under the direction of Nam Kaur Khalsa, they held the first annual Kundalini Yoga Teachers Conference, coming together to network and gain inspiration from each other, share information, and spend time with the Siri Singh Sahib. High in their priorities is to preserve the teachings that the Siri Singh Sahib has disseminated over the last 25 years. Thousands of lectures and meditations yield a treasure of information that needs preservation and organization in order to sustain the integrity of the teachings.

Khalsa International Trading

As Sikh Dharma was developing in the early years, many people started small business ventures. They needed jobs to support their families, they needed careers for the young adults to advance into, and they needed a secure source of revenue for the future growth of Sikh Dharma. With the passage of time those small businesses grew substantially and were joined together into "KIT," Khalsa International Trading. KIT is a diversified holding company, with concentrations in food manufacturing and sales, healthcare products, and service businesses. KIT provides a solid financial base for Sikh Dharma providing the sangat with independance, flexibility, and financial security.

KIT's corporate structure allows the individual business to focus on growth and innovation, while the areas of strategic and operational planning, product development, financial services, computer, and communication services are handled by specialists who are uniquely talented in their area of expertise. This gives a small business with limited resources the administrative benefits of a company many times its size.

With their feet rooted firmly in the principles of Sikh Dharma, the corporate executives of Khalsa International Trading are pioneers in progressive management techniques. Sardarni Sahiba Sopukh Kaur Khalsa is the president of Khalsa International Trading. In her insightful and intuitive way, she merges the needs of the business with the future of Sikh Dharma. Much of the research and implementation of the KIT business concept is the project of Sardarni Sahiba Siri Ram Kaur Khalsa, Chief Business Secretary. She plays an ongoing role in the process to improve teamwork and communication throughout the widespread corporation.

Akal Security, Inc., the small security company that started out with three employees, grew to become a national security service company with commercial operations in Albuquerque, Santa Fe, Los Angeles, and Houston. It expanded its focus to procuring government contracts and by the end of 1994 operated federal and state contracts in 88 cities in 14 states, employing more than 1,200 people.

Golden Temple Natural Foods had also experienced significant expansion as a major producer and distributor of granola, natural cereals, and other products. Its manufacturing plant in Eugene, Oregon, occupies 100,000 square feet with automated production lines and packaging for cereal, an expanded line of Yogi Teas, an attractive line of cosmetic oil products, and Wha Guru Chews.

The Children of Sikh Dharma Return to Amritsar

For the school year of 1994 the Sikh Dharma Foreign Education program relocated to Amritsar, the city of Guru Ram Das and the home of the hearts of the western Khalsa. Finally submerged into the Punjabi culture, the children quickly picked up the Punjabi language from their new friends and for the first time in more than 10 years, young children in white bana and bright faces could be observed doing seva at the Harimandir Sahib. They reveled in the Sikh identity that swirled around them, permeating their personalities.

Living at the Harimandir Sahib

*A*fter the devastation of 1994, I thought that we could never come with the children to live in Amritsar again. I am forever grateful for the opportunity to return and meditate at the Harimandir Sahib. For my soul it is the perfect place of healing. That is the power of the Harimandir Sahib, that it can heal so profoundly.

It is the joy, the reverence, the fervor, and the devotion of the sangat that brings sacredness to the Harimandir Sahib. When you are there, you are truly meant to be there. Its power is so real, so tangible. When you go to the Golden Temple and sit with the Guru, and with the sangat, you experience a spiritual safety because you are in your Guru's house. I have never felt the Guru like I have at the Harimandir Sahib. One day in the early morning, I heard the sound of the Guru calling my name, and He made me realize that He was calling everyone's name. All you had to do was listen.

I felt so tenderly embraced by

God and Guru that I had to be in the Harimandir Sahib every morning in the Amrit Vela. The Asa-di-Var became the vibration of my spirit and I was in ecstasy every time I sat and meditated on that divine song. It became everything to me. All I had to do was listen, and I merged in the universe. When that began to happen, I became part of the Harimandir Sahib because the sangat too was in that ecstasy. Then the sangat no longer saw me as an American, they saw me only as a daughter of the Guru.

The Golden Temple is alive and so real to me that the minute I go into meditation I can totally be there. I lived and worked there alone for eight months, and because I was there alone, the sangat took me in. They protected me, they loved me. Any Sikh who is devoted to the Guru will love any other Sikh who is devoted to the Guru. That is the blessing of being Khalsa.

Sardarni Sahiba Hari Kaur Khalsa
December 10, 1994

It had become the tradition of the western Khalsa since 1984 to commemorate the martyrdom of the Akal Takhat on the sixth of every month. It was natural for the children to continue this tradition while in India, and they proceeded to do so without hesitation. However, anything that related to the tragedy of 1984 was still a very sensitive and risky topic for the Sikhs of Amritsar, and this tradition was viewed with caution. Consistent with the political innocence of their parents, the students of SDFE moved forward with spiritual enthusiasm. Within a few months, not only did they hold a kirtan darbar on the sixth of the month, but held it at the Akal Takhat itself. As it was still in a stage of reconstruction, the children reverently sat and played kirtan at its base as the Sikhs of Amritsar and the pilgrims of the Golden Temple gathered in huge numbers to join them in honoring the sacrifice of the Akal Takhat.

The Siri Singh Sahib wrote to them: "You may ask yourself, 'Why am I here? What is all of this about?' The reality is that you are being tempered like steel. The effect of life is making you to be gem quality. When any human being is faced with a challenge and he learns to overcome that challenge, then growth is achieved.

"You may not know it, but each one of you has a special quality—something that makes you outstanding as a human being. For this reason you are in India. Through the process of life this faculty of yours will manifest and become strong. Each one of you is a leader in your own right. You have a capacity to be exceptional and to grow in ways that the average human being will not."[25]

Twenty-five Years of Sikh Dharma in the West

As 1994 came to a close, a chapter was completed for Sikh Dharma of the Western Hemisphere. Twenty-five years had passed since the man known as Yogi Bhajan came to California and first started teaching the words of Guru Nanak and the science of Kundalini Yoga. Young people picked up the banner of "Sat Nam" and soon a new generation of Khalsa emerged from every stratum of western society. Now those young Sikhs have grown and are parents with children and grandchildren of their own, looking with faith and courage toward the change of the millennium.

The Siri Singh Sahib addressed the sangat on New Years Eve, 1994, with a message of hope and upliftment. "It is my prayer that this year as you are entering into the cusp of the Age of Aquarius, where you are walking forward toward the age of knowledge, self-realization, and self-purification, you will enjoy it. Your grace and your determination will enhance and exalt you with the knowledge that you have done well.

"Serve all friends and all foes alike so that we can always say, *Wahe Guru Ji Ka Khalsa! Wahe Guru Ji Ki Fateh!* We have to earn that right. This means that purity belongs to Wahe Guru and victory belongs to Wahe Guru. It will never belong to this imaginative, defined self of today that we are passing through. God be with us all, and God be within us all, and God be around us all. Let us enjoy the sense of joy and love with the sisterhood and brotherhood of the human race. *Wahe Guru Ji Ka Khalsa! Wahe Guru Ji Ki Fateh!*"

Notes

1. Siri Guru Granth Sahibji, pg. 967

2. Yogi Bhajan; Gurdwara lecture Sept. 21, 1986

3. Yogi Bhajan; *Beads of Truth,* Winter 1987

4. Yogi Bhajan; Khalsa Council, December 1987

5. Yogi Bhajan; *Beads of Truth,* Winter 1986

6. Karta Purkh Singh Khalsa; *Beads of Truth,* Winter 1986

7. Guruka Singh Khalsa

8. Yogi Bhajan speaking at his birthday party, August 26, 1988

9. Yogi Bhajan; lecture September 26, 1988

10. Yogi Bhajan; *Identical Identity* Vol. 2, 1984

11. Yogi Bhajan; *The Power of Prayer,* 1985

12. Yogi Bhajan; *Beads of Truth,* Summer 1982

13. Yogi Bhajan; Khalsa Council, December 1990

14. Yogi Bhajan; Gurdwara Lecture, November 10, 1991

15. *Constitution of the Administrative Council of Every Sadh Sangat*

16. Siri Dharam Kaur Khalsa; *Beads of Truth,* Winter 1987

17. Shakti Parwha Kaur Khalsa; *Beads of Truth,* Summer 1985

18. Yogi Bhajan; Gurdwara lecture, November 10, 1991

19. Yogi Bhajan; Gurdwara lecture, December 31, 1994

20. Governor Bruce King; August 28, 1993

21. Representative Bill Richardson; The *Santa Fe New Mexican,* October 18, 1993

22. Attorney General Tom Udal; August 28, 1993

23. Yogi Bhajan; Gurdwara lecture, March 28, 1993

24. Yogi Bhajan; Khalsa Council, April 6, 1993

25. Yogi Bhajan in a letter to the students of SDFE, October 3, 1994

26. Yogi Bhajan from lectures in 1970 and 1984 in Los Angeles

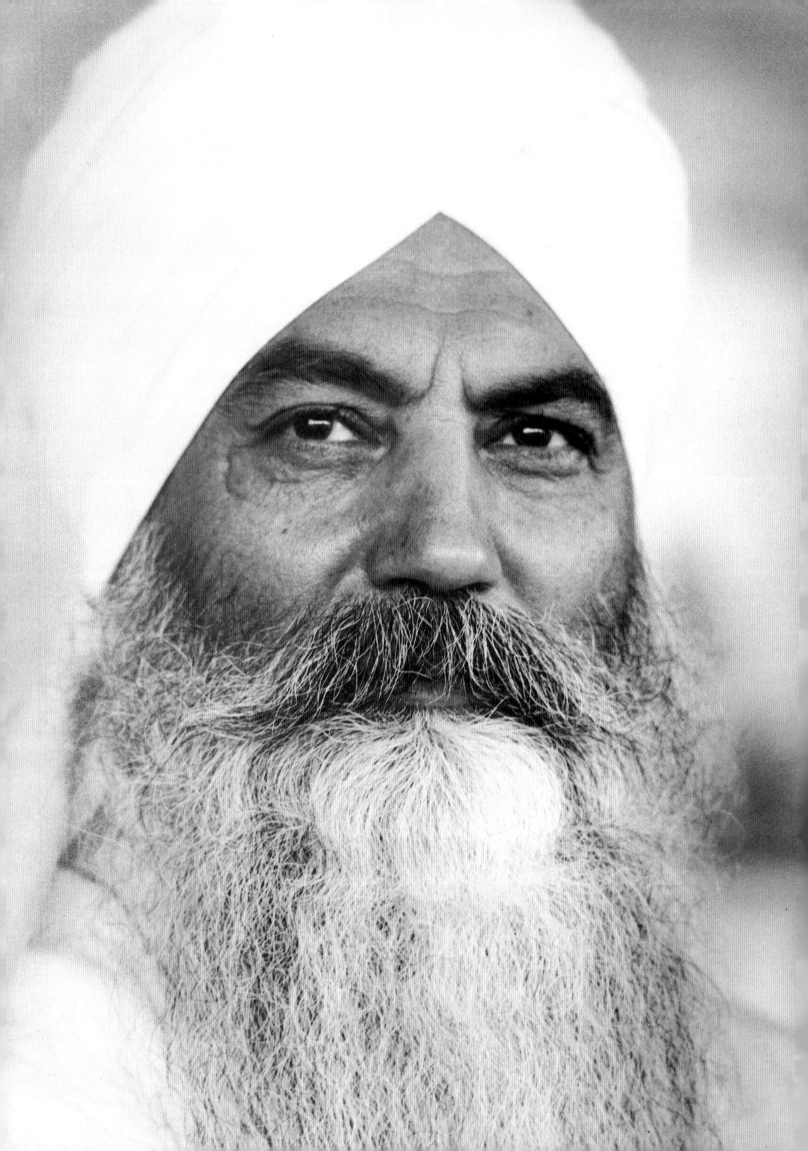

To My Students

I have given you a technical know-how: how to love each other, how to be a family. All you have to do is, with patience and with tolerance, understand each other as equals, as brothers and sisters. I came here to give you the art of togetherness. To find that Infinite God within you was my honest intention. These are the foundations that I was supposed to lay. You are a huge family now, and nobody can wipe you out. You can exist without Yogi Bhajan. Feel as free and as strong as you possibly can. Have that strength that you are all One.

This Dharma is established in the West by the Will of God, and by the Grace of Guru. Neither you nor I have played any part whatsoever. It is the destiny of the planet earth for which interrogatively, questioningly, and demonstrably the penetrating energy will prevail into the psyche, and the birth of the Khalsa shall be celebrated. It will expand, it will grow, it will establish the rule of Truth. There is nothing a human has to say or do. One day we will depart from each other forever, leaving behind a legend which will be picked up and shall be followed by those who will follow us in the time to come.

I never came here by choice. Period. I owed you a debt. To pay this debt in full, I had to leave my family, leave my country, leave all my worldly possessions. I came with nothing, and I am to go away with nothing. One last job is remaining: I am to open to you the ancient gate of wisdom. I am bound to you. I am your servant. I am not your master. [26]

Siri Singh Sahib Bhai Sahib
Harbhajan Singh Khalsa Yogiji

Glossary

Ahimsa - The principle of nonviolence.

Akal Takhat Sahib - The seat of temporal authority of the Sikhs.

Akand Path - An unbroken, continuous recitation of the *Siri Guru Granth Sahib.*

Amrit - The holy baptism of the Khalsa.

Amrit Parchar - The Amrit ceremony.

Amrit Vela - The early morning - 2:00 AM to sunrise.

Arcline - The outer layer of the auric body.

Ardas - The congregational prayer of the Sikhs.

Asa Di Var - A long, heroic composition including the words of Guru Nanak, Guru Angad, and Guru Ram Das. Traditional sung in the early morning.

Ashram - Spiritual center.

Aura and Auric Body - The electromagnetic field around an object or living thing.

Banis - The daily prayers of the Sikhs.

Bhog Ceremony - The ceremony celebrating the end of an Akand Path.

Chakra - Energy centers within the body.

Chauree Sahib - The horsehair fan that is waved in reverence over the *Siri Guru Granth Sahib.*

Cherdi Kala - The exalted rising of the spirit.

Churidas - Traditional Sikh leggings.

Darbar - The court of a king or a guru.

Darbar Sahib - The Golden Temple in Amritsar.

Darshan - The blessed sight of a saint, sage, or holy man.

Das Vand - The giving of one-tenth of your earnings to the religious community fund.

Dasam Granth - The compiled writings of Guru Gobind Singh

Gatka - The martial art of sword play as developed by the Sikhs.

Golden Temple - The Harimandir Sahib in Amritsar, the Sikhs most revered temple.

Granthi - The person who performs the priestly duties in a gurdwara

Grisht Ashram - The life of a householder.

Gurbani Kirtan - The verses of the *Siri Guru Granth Sahib* and other holy writings sung in melody.

Gurdwara - The Sikh religious service, also a Sikh temple.

Gurmat - The knowledge of the Sikh technology and history

Gurmukhi - The language of *Siri Guru Granth Sahib* created by Guru Angad.

Gurpurb - A Sikh religious holy day.

Gursikh - A Sikh of the Guru.

Guru - Literally, one who takes you from darkness to light, a teacher of spiritual wisdom.

Harimandir Sahib - The Golden Temple in Amritsar.

Hukam - The order from God, the will of God. When the *Siri Guru Granth Sahib* is opened for guidance, the words that are read are the Hukam.

Jaap Sahib - A composition of Guru Gobind Singh. One of the daily prayers of the Sikhs.

Japji Sahib - The primary composition of Guru Nanak. One of the daily prayers of the Sikhs.

Jatha - A group.

Jathadar - A group leader.

Kachera - Sikh underwear. One of the five required accoutrements of a Khalsa Sikh.

Kandha - The double-edged sword.

Kanga - A small comb worn in the hair. One of the five required accoutrements of a Khalsa Sikh.

Kar Seva - Volunteer work.

Kara - A steel bangle. One of the five required accoutrements of a Khalsa Sikh.

Kesh, Keshas - Long, uncut hair. One of the five required accoutrements of a Khalsa Sikh.

Kinesiology - The medical art of pressure points.

Kirpan - A Sikh dagger or knife. One of the five required accoutrements of a Khalsa Sikh.

Kirtan - devotional music in praise of God.

Kirtan Jatha - A group of musicians who play Gurbani Kirtan

Kirtanis - musicians in a kirtan jatha

KRI - Kundalini Research Institute

Kriyas - A yogic exercise that incorporates hand and eye position, breath, meditation, and mantra.

Kundal - Coil, literally "the coil of the beloved's hair."

Kurta - Indian-style tunic

Langar - Blessed food served following a gurdwara service.

Lavan - The composition of Guru Ram Das sung at the Sikh wedding ceremony.

Mahan Tantric - The living teacher of White Tantric Yoga.

Mala - Meditation beads.

Mugal - The occupying Islamic forces in pre-British India.

Naad - The science and technology of the sound current.

Nihung - A Sikh who considers himself to be part of Guru Gobind Singh's army, wearing the dress of a warrior, living a life of discipline, and bearing arms at all times.

Nitnem - A book containing the daily prayers of the Sikhs.

Paath - Recitation of the daily prayers of the Sikhs.

Palki Sahib - The dais on which the *Siri Guru Granth Sahib* is placed.

Panth - The Sikh nation.

Panth Khalsa -The Khalsa Nation.

Parkarma - The walkway around a temple.

Prashad - The sweet, holy food served after Ardas and Hukam in a Sikh gurdwara service.

Punj Piare - The five Beloved Ones of Guru Gobind Singh.

Rehiras - The evening daily prayer of the Sikhs.

Rehit - Form and discipline of the Khalsa. Rehit Maryada is the code of conduct of that discipline.

Rumalas - The cloths laid around the *Siri Guru Granth Sahib.*

Sadh Sangat - A gathering of the disciplined ones.

Sadhana - Daily spiritual practice.

Sahaj Yoga - The effortless merger with the One.

Sangat - The body of the congregation.

Sant Supai - One who blends the attributes of a soldier and a saint.

Saropa - A cloth that is presented in the presence of the Sangat and the *Siri Guru Granth Sahib* as a symbol of honor.

Sarovar - The blessed tank of water surrounding the Harimandir Sahib.

Seva - Selfless service.

Sevadar - One who performs selfless service.

Shabad - The Word of God. The teachings of the *Siri Guru Granth Sahib.*

Shakti - Spiritual power.

Shanti - Peace.

Shiromani Akali Dal - The political party of the Sikhs.

Shiromani Gurdwara Parbandhak Committee - The chief administrative body for the Sikhs.

Sidh Gosht - The composition of Guru Nanak when he addresses the Yogis.

Siri Guru Granth Sahib - The living Guru of the Sikhs.

Siri Sahib - A blessed sword.

Sukhmani Sahib - A composition of Guru Arjun Dev.

Tabla - Indian drums.

Yatra - A spiritual journey.

Yatri - People on a spiritual journey.

Captions & Photo Credits

Page 53. *Siri Singh Sahib Bhai Sahib Harbhajan Singh Khalsa Yogiji offering Ardas during Khalsa Council 1985.* Photo: Soorya Kaur Khalsa.

Page 54. *Yogi Bhajan teaching in Northern California in August, 1970.* Photo: Sikh Dharma Archives.

Page 55. *Yogi Bhajan enjoys a rare, solitary moment during a teaching tour in October, 1970.* Photo: Sikh Dharma Archives.

Pages 56–57. *Yogi Bhajan teaching at the Guru Ram Das Ashram on Melrose Ave, Los Angeles in August, 1969. This ashram, the converted garage of Jules Buccieri's antique store, was the first Guru Ram Das Ashram in the West.* Photo: Sikh Dharma Archives.

Page 58. *Siri Singh Sahib Harbhajan Singh Khalsa Yogiji, Española, New Mexico, 1987.* Photo: Soorya Kaur Khalsa.

Page 59. *Above left, Sardar Ranbir Singh and Sardar Kulbir Singh, 1980.* Photo:

Soorya Kaur Khalsa. *Above right, Bibiji Inderjit Kaur, Bhai Sahiba of Sikh Dharma, 1993.* Photo: Sikh Dharma Archives. *Below, Yogi Bhajan playfully teases his daughter, Kamaljit Kaur Kohli, 1985.* Photo: Soorya Kaur Khalsa. *Not shown are Ranbir Singh's wife, Dr. Avneesh Kaur and their three sons, Angad Singh, Fateh Singh, and Sahib Singh. Also not shown are Kamaljit Kaur's husband, Sat Pal Singh Kohli and their two daughters, Kamal Charan Kaur and Taran Jeet Kaur.*

Pages 60–61. *M.S.S. Krishna Kaur Khalsa and Sat Purkha Singh meditating during a White Tantric Yoga kriya at Summer Solstice Sadhana, 1985, New Mexico.* Photo: Soorya Kaur Khalsa.

Page 62. *White Tantric Yoga at Summer Solstice Sadhana, 1985, New Mexico.* Photo: Soorya Kaur Khalsa.

Page 63. *Above, S.S. Subagh Singh Khalsa and S.S. Subagh Kaur Khalsa walk together during a break in the White Tantric*

Yoga meditation during Summer Solstice Sadhana, 1986. Photo: Soorya Kaur Khalsa. *Below, participants of Summer Solstice Sadhana, 1984, keep up during a Kundalini Yoga class.* Photo: Soorya Kaur Khalsa.

Pages 64–65. *Lines of people in the fields of Ram Das Puri during the blind-walk meditation at Summer Solstice Sadhana, 1985, New Mexico.* Photo: Soorya Kaur Khalsa.

Page 66. *Morning Sadhana meditations, led by M.S.S. Ram Das Singh Khalsa and Guru Trang Singh Khalsa, Summer Solstice Sadhana, 1980, New Mexico.* Photo: Sikh Dharma Archives.

Page 67. *Guru Meher Singh Khalsa receives the holy Amrit during the Amrit Ceremony at Summer Solstice Sadhana, 1985. The Sikh baptism of Amrit initiates the Sikh into the order of the Khalsa.* Photo: Soorya Kaur Khalsa.

Pages 68–69. *The Siri Singh Sahib founded Peace Prayer Day in 1985 to pray for world peace and for peace in the individual soul. This annual event of the 3HO Foundation draws thousands of people each year to pray together at the beautiful mountain site of Ram Das Puri in New Mexico.* Photo: Sat Simran Kaur Khalsa.

Page 70. *Students of the Sikh Dharma Foreign Education Program stand in parade during a program at Sant Singh Sukha Singh School in Amritsar in 1995.* Photo: Soorya Kaur Khalsa.

Page 71. *The Siri Singh Sahib lectures during Khalsa Women's Training Camp in 1988. KWTC is a five-week, spiritual camp for women held at Hacienda de Guru Ram Das in Española, New Mexico.* Photo: Soorya Kaur Khalsa.

Page 72. *Gurujeet Kaur Khalsa and Gurbani Kaur Khalsa of Española share the sisterhood of Khalsa Women's Training Camp in 1986 with their young children.* Photo: Soorya Kaur Khalsa.

Page 73. *Women meditate together at Khalsa Women's Training Camp.* Photo: Soorya Kaur Khalsa.

Page 74. *The Siri Singh Sahib spends a spontaneous and relaxed morning with guests at his ranch in New Mexico in 1987.* Photo: Soorya Kaur Khalsa.

Page 75. *The Siri Singh Sahib and Bibiji stand together.* Photo: Soorya Kaur Khalsa.

Page 76. *Jagat Guru Singh Khalsa and Gurudev Kaur Khalsa sit together during their wedding ceremony in 1994.* Photo: Shanti Kaur Khalsa.

Page 77. *Siri Mukta Singh Khalsa and Fateh Kaur Khalsa are married in the Gurdwara at Hacienda de Guru Ram Das in New Mexico in 1994.* Photo: Soorya Kaur Khalsa.

Page 78. *Long, uncut hair, known as* kesh, *and the Sikh dagger, known as* kirpan, *are two of the five characteristics of the Khalsa Rehit. 1979* Photo: Soorya Kaur Khalsa.

Page 79. *During the winter of 1982, the young boys of the Sikh Dharma Foreign*

Education program stayed with Baba Nihal Singh and toured the Punjab giving gatka and kirtan programs. Photo: Sikh Dharma Archives.

Page 80. *Sant Baba Joginder Singh Moni of Hazoor Sahib Gurdwara presents saropas to the Siri Singh Sahib, Bibiji, and Kulbir Singh during KWTC, 1986.* Photo: Sat Simran Kaur Khalsa.

Page 81. *The Siri Singh Sahib and Baba Nihal Singh embrace in an emotional reunion in 1987. This was their first meeting since the tragedy in Amritsar in 1984.* Photo: Soorya Kaur Khalsa.

Page 82. *The Siri Singh Sahib on a teaching tour in France in 1986.* Photo: Soorya Kaur Khalsa.

Page 83. *The Siri Singh Sahib meets with Pope John Paul II in Rome.* Photo: Sikh Dharma Archives.

Page 84. *Above, the Siri Singh Sahib talks with President Bill Clinton during a fundraiser in Albuquerque, New Mexico in the 1992 elections.* Photo: Sikh Dharma Archives. *Below, The Siri Singh is the friend and confidant of many state leaders in New Mexico. From left to right: Attorney General Tom Udal, US Representative Bill Richardson, Siri Singh Sahib, Earl Potter, and Jill Cooper. 1991* Photo: Soorya Kaur Khalsa.

Page 85. *The Siri Singh Sahib has met with the Dalai Lama, the leader of the Tibetan Buddhists, several times over the past 25 years. There is a bond of friend-*

ship and support between their two peoples. 1979 Photo: Sat Simram Kaur Khalsa.

Page 86. *The Siri Singh Sahib confers with the Prime Minister of India, P.V. Narasimha Rao in 1993.* Photo: Harbhajan Singh Longman, Longman Studios, New Delhi, India.

Page 87. *"Holy man among diplomats," the Siri Singh Sahib enjoys meeting with Minister of Parliament, S. Surendrajeet Singh Aluwalia and the late former President of India, Giani Zail Singh in 1993.* Photo: Harbhajan Singh Longman, Longman Studios, New Delhi, India.

Pages 88–89. *The Siri Singh Sahib addresses the sangat during a gurdwara held at the home of M.P. Surendrajeet Singh Aluwalia in 1993.* Photo: Soorya Kaur Khalsa.

Page 90. *The Siri Singh Sahib speaks briefly to the crowd during a train stop in Ambala during his 1993 tour of the Punjab.* Photo: Harbhajan Singh Longman, Longman Studios, New Delhi, India.

Page 91. *The citizens of the city of Amritsar extend a warm welcome to the Siri Singh Sahib and the western Sikhs during their 1995 visit to India.* Photo: Soorya Kaur Khalsa.

Pages 92–93. *Students from Sikh Dharma Foreign Education program play Gurbani Kirtan at Bangla Sahib Gurdwara in New Delhi in 1993. From left to right: Sat Kartar Kaur Khalsa, Sat Bachan Kaur Khalsa, Sat Pavan Kaur Khalsa, Sat Mittar Kaur Khalsa, Harimandir Jot Singh Khalsa.* Photo: Soorya Kaur Khalsa.

Page 94. *S.S. Pritpal Singh Khalsa and his son, Sat Pal Singh Khalsa, during a visit to India in 1995.* Photo: Soorya Kaur Khalsa.

Page 95. *Sikhs from the Sikh Dharma Foreign Education program meditate at the Golden Temple in 1995. From left to right: Mahan Kirn Kaur Khalsa, Sat Hari Kaur Khalsa, Siri Sundri Kaur Khalsa, Guru Mustak Singh Khalsa, and, sitting in front of the group, Guru Amrit Hari Kaur Khalsa.* Photo: Soorya Kaur Khalsa.

Page 96. *S.S. Jot Singh Khalsa of Khalsa Kirpans grinds a knife blade in his workshop in Massachusetts.* Photo: Soorya Kaur Khalsa.

Page 97 *The artwork of Khalsa Kirpans take their place amongst the museum quality swords and kirpans of the Sikh Dharma Archives. 1995* Photo: Anton Brkic, Anton's Studio, Santa Fe, New Mexico.

Pages 98–99 *The beautiful, artistic jewelry, in precious and semiprecious stones, adorn the Sikh Dharma Archives as the "crown jewels" of Sikh Dharma of the Western Hemisphere. 1995* Photo: Anton Brkic, Anton's Studio, Santa Fe, New Mexico.

Page 100. *Handwritten and illustrated copies of the* Siri Guru Granth Sahib, *priceless and irreplaceable, are lovingly preserved in the Sikh Dharma Archives. 1995* Photo: Anton Brkic, Anton's Studio, Santa Fe, New Mexico